# What People Are Saying

"I was there on stage with Bonnie when it became apparent that something just wasn't right. That night, after a visit to the hospital, I wondered what could possibly be happening? After Bonnie's MS diagnosis, I observed an admirable strength and determination that was truly a thing of beauty to behold. She used her incredible energy to overcome, and fight a battle that she refused to lose. She came back strong, wrote new songs and resumed her singing career. Her book tells her story. It's a story where every page is worth reading."

Jerry Jacobs - F.A.B. Company


"Unique, interesting, a real life story."

Dr. Roger M Bagg


"Humor. Warmth. Personality. "Take Time" to read this personal, informative book."

Kellie S. Fitzsimmons, B.S.N., R.N.


"Bonnie was my performing partner and friend before, during, and after her attack of MS. She represents the kind of courage we would all like to have. She became determined not to be beaten by this ugly disease and she won. She has a daughter, is still driven and hard working and her book is inspirational to all of us, those with MS and those without. I am proud to be her friend."

Ralph Achilles, F.A.B. Company
from THE FUNNY ONE
visit me at ralphachilles.net


"One of Bonnie's real strengths as a friend, parent, performer and now author is her delightful sense of humor. Her smiles and hearty laughs come easy and often – sometimes with a wink and a mischievous but charming side glance. That's tough to do in print, but she's done it in her new book."

# MS Entertainer

## Rodeo, Music, and Multiple Sclerosis

## Bonnie Lynne Ellison

Photograpy by Ted Lemke
Stage Lights by Ken Williams;
Illustrations by Bennet Evans

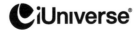

MS ENTERTAINER
Rodeo, Music, and Multiple Sclerosis

iUniverse books may be ordered through booksellers or by contacting:

iUniverse
1663 Liberty Drive
Bloomington, IN 47403
www.iuniverse.com
1-800-Authors (1-800-288-4677)

Because of the dynamic nature of the Internet, any Web addresses or links contained in this book may have changed since publication and may no longer be valid. The views expressed in this work are solely those of the author and do not necessarily reflect the views of the publisher, and the publisher hereby disclaims any responsibility for them.

ISBN: 978-1-4502-4256-1 (sc)
ISBN: 978-1-4502-4257-8 (e)

Print information available on the last page.

iUniverse rev. date: 06/10/2019

*To Sophie and Savannah*

*To my family and friends*
*who inspired and guided me*
*Thank you.*

*Special Thanks to*
*Ann, Ted, Pat, and Frank*

*Thank you Achilles and Frank for gracing*
*my book with your songs.*

# Contents

# MS ENTERTAINER Songs
## All Rights Reserved

*Introduction: "Y'All Put Your Shoes On" (➤ 1977 Bonnie Lynne Ellison)*

*I "I Never Made It in The 50's" (➤ 1975 Francis E. Bruen)*
   *"Fly High" (➤ 1972 Bonnie Lynne Ellison)*
*II "Worth the Time" (➤ 1975 Ralph Achilles)*
*III "Look at Me" (➤ 2002 Bonnie Lynne Ellison)*
*IV "I Can't Love You Enough" (➤ 1972 Bonnie Lynne Ellison)*
   *"Easy Lovin' Day" (➤ 1972 Bonnie Lynne Ellison)*
   *"Love Me 'til the Rain Goes Away" (➤ 1973 Ralph Achilles)*
*V "The Two Peddler Men" (➤ 1966 Ralph Achilles)*
*VI "Stick It" (➤ 1975 Francis E. Bruen)*
   *"Flower Power Petal Pusher" (➤ 1970 Bonnie Lynne Ellison)*
*VII "Hank's Raisin' Hell in Heaven" (➤ 2005 Bonnie Lynne Ellison)*
   *"Watermelon Is a King's Delight" (➤ 1966 Ralph Achilles)*
*VIII "We Live As We Can" (➤ 1982 Bonnie Lynne Ellison)*
*IX "Sorry, We're Closed" (➤ 1977 Bonnie Lynne Ellison)*
*X "The Night Belongs to the Entertainer" (➤ 1970 Ralph Achilles)*
   *"Take Time" (➤ 1973 Bonnie Lynne Ellison)*
*XI "I'm a Star" (➤ 1973 Bonnie Lynne Ellison)*
*XII "Life Is Just A Puff Of Dreams" (➤ 1973 Ralph Achilles)*

*Reflections: "Good Lovin' Man" (➤ 2001 Bonnie Lynne Ellison)*
   *"Colorado Sky" (➤ 1966 Ralph Achilles)*

# Acknowledgments

Forgive me for not acknowledging individuals separately. There are too many. I sincerely thank everyone who has contributed their time, patience, and energy to make this book possible. Thank you, Bob, for suggesting that I keep a diary about my MS. I could never have remembered.

# *Y'All Put Your Shoes On*

*Early mornin' sunlight shinin'... On my bed.*
*Early mornin' rooster crowin'... In my head.*
*Early mornin' breakfast smells... Bacon and eggs.*
*Momma's callin' up the stairs... "Y'all shake a leg!"*

*Us kids washin' up, gettin' to the table,*
*Fightin" for our favorite seats.*
*Papa offers the blessin',*
*Thank God we've got enough to eat.*

*How come I've always got to be the one,*
*Shuckin' corn and shellin' peas?*
*Ain't nothing like momma's cookin',*
*Momma always aims to please.*

*There ain't a lot happenin',*
*When you're twenty-five miles from town.*
*And the nearest house is cousin Billy's,*
*Five miles down.*

*The days get long, and us kids fight,*
*Everybody's waitin' for the sound...*
*"Y'all put your shoes on,*
*We're gonna go to town!"*

*Mama's in her curlers, us kids in the back of the truck.*
*Pappa's at the wheel, thinkin' bout rain, prayin' for a little luck.*
*John Wayne's punchin' cowboys, in town at the picture show.*
*Someday I'm gonna be like him, leave the weeds in the garden to grow.*

*chorus:*

*Now I'm the momma and you're the pappa, on the porch in the rockin' chair,*
*And we've got kids of our own now, just breathin' that country air.*
*You're pappa, he don't say much, reads the newspaper with a frown.*
*I'm stitchin' up britches while the kids are playin', with the dog in the dirt on the*
*ground.*

*chorus:*

*But your daddy knows what to do when the lonesome country blues start*
*gettin' us down.*
*(He says) "Y'all put your shoes on,*
*We're gonna go to town!"*

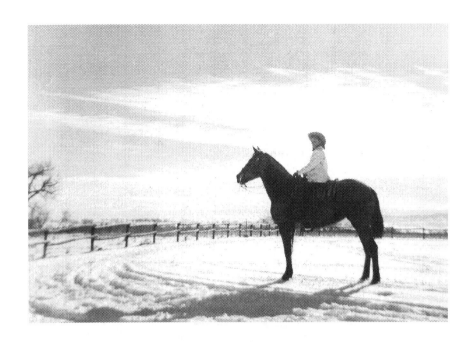

# Introduction
## August, 1964

"I love the rodeo."

"Number 821," the megaphone called to contestants, through the dusty, afternoon 90° heat of the National Little Britches Rodeo Finals. Adrenaline rushed through my body, as I lightly touched Lady with my spurs. I was ready to go!

Unfortunately, I was the only one... My tan buckskin mare refused to move. I repeated my spur therapy, with a more serious jab this time. My horse backed up to clearly emphasize her point.

"Number 821," was repeated again. Anxious and embarrassed, I looked around to see who was watching. Determined to show her who was the boss, I jabbed my spurs into the sides of her body.

I felt the horse gather her hind legs under her, withdraw, and then stand straight up, actually launching me into heaven, before she began to fall backwards...on top of me. Like a pro... I rode her to the ground...

Lady was a big girl...1500 pounds of muscle and determination.

I was a sixteen year old brown-eyed, brown-haired girl…120 pounds of "no fear," and full of determination to win the National Little Britches Rodeo Championship Saddle. We each had a mind of our own… Unfortunately, my horse also had 1500 pounds to accomplish her desires. I was seriously outweighed.

Little Britches was a rodeo held for kids from eight to eighteen years old. The National Finals were held in my hometown, Littleton, Colorado, at the Arapahoe County Fairgrounds.

Forrest Hammes and Varian Ashbaugh founded the Junior rodeo in 1952 with events ranging from the Queen Contest and Barrel Racing, to Bareback, Saddle Bronc, and Bull Riding. The non-profit organization continued through 1978 before moving to Colorado Springs. Under Forrest's direction, as the Secretary of The Colorado Fair Association, Little Britches grew to ninety-nine rodeos nationwide, from California to New York, was host to many political and legal dignitaries, and was televised nationally.

Even before Little Britches, I developed an "irresistible urge" to own a horse. Maybe I had inherited it. I was born at the Colonial Stables, an English Riding and Jumping Academy, which my father managed in Baltimore, Maryland, before we moved into the city, where he worked for Martin Marietta (Lockheed Martin), a national aerospace defense company.

I can remember secretly wishing for a pony every year before blowing my birthday candles out. The walls of my room were covered with horse pictures. I used to dream that on Christmas morning, I'd wake up, and there would be no presents under the tree. But when I was told to go outside, there was a pony tied to our front door.

Prayers do work! But it wasn't a pony, and he didn't get to live in our suburban back yard behind our inter-city row houses.

In junior high, my father was transferred from Baltimore, Maryland, to Denver, Colorado and I was transformed from an "eastern city slicker" into a western cowgirl. My dreams came true. I got a horse and learned to ride western style, like the cowboys do…

When I opened my eyes, I was laying in the dirt, surrounded by adult cowboys, jeans, cowboy boots, hats and paramedics, with a stretcher.

"Don't move! Don't move! What hurts?" they repeated. Waking up, with the help of smelling salts, I was relieved that my horse was standing close by. At least she was all right.

My leg hurt, but in an attempt not to worry my mother, who was watching from the grandstand, I said, "I'm all right." But they persisted. "Don't move!" Feeling incapable... I agreed. They carefully lifted me on to the stretcher.

"Give the little lady a hand," the announcer suggested as they carried me in front of the grandstand, towards the First Aid Station. I raised my arm, acknowledging the audience's support, and to show mom that I was still alive. I'm a born entertainer. I love the applause...

Once inside, doctors immediately cut open my Levi jean pants from my waist down to my Justin boot to reveal a multi-colored left leg, still attached to a very multi-colored thigh...a sort of rainbow effect.

One look by all, and I was carried directly into the ambulance... x-rays were a necessity. I'd been lucky so far. I'd never broken a bone before, although, my head had taken quite a battering through the years.

Now, I was scared. I felt like I was going to throw up...I could feel my nerves tingling throughout my body, and even "inside" my stomach. I just knew that I'd broken something this time! My emergency doctors seemed to agree. They thought it was my upper left thigh bone. I felt sick remembering painful stories that I'd heard about resetting broken bones. Why couldn't I start with a little bone, not the largest one in my leg?

This was a first. I'd never ridden in an ambulance before. At least, I was the center of sound and attention. But I hurt, and my biggest fear was that my pain was just beginning. Ambulances are very sterile, antiseptic. And this trip seemed way too sterile, for this rodeo rider!

The ambulance pulled into the doctor's office, and I was motionlessly taken into the x-ray machine. Pictures were taken, and

I was moved to a waiting room, allowing the doctor time to examine my film results. I was left alone, in fear, to wait... and to think...

My dad, Merton Bagg, was the horseman in our family. He always appeared taller than five foot seven due to his tan Stetson hat. He always appeared strong to me, because of his athletic ability. He always was successful because he had "heart." He will always be my John Wayne replica with a harsh, demanding voice, sarcastic humor, a soft heart, and a love for animals. He always said that I could ride, and hold on, as well as anyone. His philosophy was: "When problems start showin', hitch up your buckle, and keep on goin'... " Dad and I were competitors. We were tough! And we were winners! Good was never good enough. I could always do better...

Dr. Frank Martaurano, our Italian family rodeo doctor just kept patching me up, asking, "When are you going to stop?"

My fragile mother worried about my horse participation. Maybe it was because she had broken her back as a young woman when she got bucked off of a rental horse. Maybe it was because I had ridden a run away horse "through" a fence. Or maybe, she worried about the "blood clot" I had gotten on my head, after being bucked off another one of our horses. Or maybe her fear stemmed from the Wild Horse Bareback Bronc competition I'd been in, when I pulled the bareback riggin' over the horse's head, and was thrown to the ground breathless. Mom just wasn't a competitor...

Dr. Martaurano finally appeared. Thankfully, he had good news. Nothing was broken... Only "badly bruised." I guess so... 1500 pounds of "bruising." I felt more "crushed" than "bruised."

My mom, Vivian Lucille Bagg, was the nurse in our family, five and a half feet with thick, black, wavy hair and deep black eyes of mercy. She took me home. We hobbled into the bedroom, together, where she proceeded to take off my other boot. ("A good cowboy never goes to bed with his boots on.") This boot removable was an impossible job. Perseverance and strength failed repeatedly until finally, she succeeded, and the boot came off.

My right ankle and foot were both swollen twice their normal size, and were also quite colorful. And this was my good side! No one had looked at my right side. I had said that my left leg hurt. So, it was back to the doctors for more x-rays. Maybe, I had still broken something!

Dr. Martaurano's final report was a "badly sprained right ankle, a badly bruised left leg, multiple bruises, pulled tendons, squashed muscles," you name it, two injured feet and two injured legs. I got wrapped up, and was given a cane to maneuver.

I knew I was "tough," but two "crushed" legs and a cane were no replacement for a saddle. I had followed the Little Britches Rodeo circuit all year, accumulating event-winning points. This was not the time for my championship horse to refuse an event. This was not good for my "National reputation." However, this seemed to be a necessary time for my recuperation...

Winning was easy for me. My athletic abilities allowed me to graduate from holding the record at North Elementary School in the Girl's Softball Throw, to bowling on television in "Pin Busters," to winning the Vocal Music Award at Grant Junior High School, to winning ribbons, trophies, and buckles in the Little Britches Rodeo, to winning national competitions in the Kiwanis Club Stars of Tomorrow Talent Show for singing with my guitar (just like Judy Collins).

I climbed the ladder... from softball, to rodeo, to singing. I loved the applause, from rodeo fans, to talent show audience, to auditoriums and concerts. I took guitar lessons, and found that I could play music by ear. It was easy! No effort! It was natural. Music was my passion! I loved to sing, and I loved to perform!

As time went by, I changed from the rodeo circuit to the entertainment circuit. Mom was relieved, perceiving performing as less dangerous. (What was she thinking?) It wasn't easy, but I proved her wrong!

# I NEVER MADE IT IN THE 50'S

*Chorus:*

> I never made it in the fifties, ...
> And I probably won't make it now, ...
> But I'll keep singin' my songs, ...anyhow

*Verse 1*

> I was there when they first did bee bop-a loo
> And everybody did the stroll,
> 'And long tall Sally was the queen, ...of rock 'n roll

*Bridge:*

> Now everbody's looking back (Aaaah)
> It's like a train fallin' off the track (Aaaah)
> Tryin' to get something back (Aaaah)
> It ain't nothin' but an act, (aaaah)
> Cause yesterday's gone.

*Verse 2*

> I can't tell 'em what they wanna hear
> I got to tell 'em what's on my mind,
> If they don't wanna buy it, ... I guess that's fine

*Chorus:*

> I never made it in the fifties, . . .
> And I probably won't make it now, ...
> But I'll keep singin' my songs, ...anyhow

9 years later…

# I

## First Month

## November, 1973

"It's the water…and a lot more…" At least that's what the Olympia Brewing Company claims. I had never been to Olympia before, although I had been in Washington State. But this was the first time that I had ever been in a city which shared it's name with a brewery. I wasn't actually much of a beer drinker at twenty-five. But being from Colorado, I had been known to taste a Coors on special occasions. And since I was in Olympia, I was now interested in their special water. Coors beer is supposedly brewed with pure Rocky Mountain Spring Water, while Olympia is made with Artesian water. I naturally realized the necessity of a taste comparison. After drinking some of each, for tasting purposes, I only realized that it is very difficult to distinguish Artesian from spring water. I guess that's why it takes "a lot more" in Olympia.

What they should have said was: It's the water… and a lot more… water. It had been raining since I had arrived. All sightseeing trips had been postponed due to the weather, which wasn't cooperating to offer much of an Olympia welcoming. It was gloomy, cloudy, and very wet. The clouds took away the sun; the rain constantly drizzled.

While the weather outside was depressing, I was in Olympia trying to keep the depression outside. At least, that was supposed to be my job… I was a twenty-five year old professional, performing at the Evergreen Inn with my two partners, Frank Bruen and Jerry Jacobs. Our group, the F. A. B. Company, did a quiet show using acoustical instruments while emphasizing our original songs and comedy.

The Evergreen lounge appeared warm and intimate. There was a high ceiling with two walls made entirely out of glass. Very classy... The inn was situated on a hill with windows overlooking a bay. The motel which adjoined it offered a touch of elegance with shops of every kind, everything from a beauty shop, barber shop, and gift shop, to a laundry service, banquet and dining rooms, and oversized bathtubs in each room, which could be more easily recognized as small private indoor pools.

Outside, everything was green... Green trees grew right out of the green grass. Coming from Colorado in November, there were no leaves on the trees and the grass was still brown. At that time of year, winter is very apparent. But I had left the ice and snow behind for all of this Olympian green.

Colorado is very dry and I soon discovered that Washington is very wet. It continued to rain for the next three weeks while I was there. In Colorado, a nice rain shower or thunderstorm is always welcome. But this continuous, humid, damp, cloudy, drizzly, depressive weather was something new for me.

While it kept raining outside, we kept waiting inside for the weather to clear. That was a mistake. I ended up seeing a great deal of the stage and the inside of my motel, and very little of Olympia. I even missed the highlight of my trip...the brewery tour.

We'd been in Washington for about two and one-half weeks. The rain was now affecting us all, getting us down. I didn't have a car. I had ridden up with Jerry on this trip. I could have used his car, but I didn't ask very often. Rain looks generally the same wherever you are.

We did go skiing one day. Being from Colorado, ski country U.S.A., we were all very disappointed with the snow conditions. Slush conditions would be a better description. It was the first time I had ever been at the base of the ski slope when it was raining...

Snow or sleet or whatever it was, was coming down hard. It was one of those fogged-up goggles, can't see days, on the slopes. Whatever was coming, one thing was for sure: it was wet! And it wasn't the only one. I was soaked! In my Colorado ski attire of long underwear, jeans, sweaters, ski jacket, gloves and hat, I became a dripping icicle.

Being wet, the snow on the ground was also very heavy. This again was not like the powder dry Colorado skiing conditions. I was down in the snow and back up so many times that day, I finally just wanted to give up and stay down. I was exhausted… and embarrassed.

This was the first time that I had ever skied with Jerry. All of the way, driving up to the slopes, we had anxiously talked about skiing. Not being one to undersell myself, there seemed to be a great deal of distance between my car conversation and my exhibited skiing ability. Jerry, in his understanding manner, helped me make excuses for my poor demonstration on the slopes. I even managed a new trick on this trip. I dropped my ski pole from the chair lift…

Everyone has a bad day occasionally, but these days in Olympia, everything seemed to be going wrong. You might say that I got up on the wrong side of the bed. But that's actually an understatement, for I had noticed during the last few days, strange feelings when I did get up. For instance, when the motel operator gave me a wake up call, I'd jump out of bed to answer the phone feeling dizzy or faint, and bumping into things, as if I were drunk. But, being a woman, these lightheaded sensations were not totally unusual to me during certain times of the month. I attributed my carelessness to being startled by the phone and my clumsiness to my overanxious response. I didn't think very much about it at the time.

I never recognized any possible connection between my wake up feeling and my leg. It had also been acting strange lately. It felt heavy. It may sound funny, but I told Frank and Jerry that my right leg felt heavy. As part of my on the road activities, I'd been exercising daily in the privacy of my motel room. I found nothing noticeably wrong with my leg. It moved normally and didn't feel numb, but it was heavy… Maybe I was just imagining it… convincing myself that it was heavy. Maybe it was all in my head…

Imagined or not, my leg seemed to be getting heavier over the next few days, until I began to slightly limp when walking. I thought that I disguised it well though. Nothing seemed obvious; it was my own little secret. Or, at least I thought so until someone asked me what was wrong with my leg. My secret was evidently obvious. But my answer to the question was not. I finally casually responded with, "I only turned my ankle."

I don't lie very often. Anyway, this was not a complete lie. For, lately, I had turned my ankle over several times. But if you could only have seen the height of the boxy heels that were on my new shoes, turning my ankle wouldn't be a surprise. I hadn't worn the shoes very long, and I was having trouble with them. Anyway, my natural athletic abilities always superceded my gracefulness. I promised myself that I would slow down and concentrate on the latter.

My husband called me on our third anniversary. I had just received a dozen long stemmed red roses from him. I was content and very much in love… When I spoke to him, I didn't mention anything about my limping. It didn't seem appropriate for our conversation at the time. I had decided to make an appointment to see a doctor and I didn't think there was anything that Bob could do for me half way across the United States.

The day after my roses arrived, I jumped out of bed to answer my morning wake-up call, ran into the dresser, and barely saved my flowers from falling to the floor. That's all I would have needed. I realized that getting from the bed to the phone was becoming more of a challenge than I was interested in.

That same day I decided to try my father's old football remedy for leg injuries, "Walk it out!" I went Christmas shopping with Jerry and his girl at a shopping center with a large enclosed mall, offering me a lot of walking space. But after dad's remedy didn't seem to work very well, I decided to call a medical clinic. I was frustrated with my new condition, to say the least. My leg worked perfectly well, but felt heavy. And then my ankle also occasionally turned over. I wasn't sure who to call or who to ask for. What kind of doctor handles heavy legs?

The closest phone was outside of the mall. I was angry and frustrated, but determined to find out what exactly was wrong with me. I limped over to the phone, laid my purse down, and got my wallet out. It was damp and cold. I was so cold, my hands were shaking. I got my only dime out, dropped it, and then began to hunt on the ground. Fortunately, it hadn't gone far.

I called information and asked for the closest medical center to the motel where I was staying. I then called the number, explained to the receptionist that my foot turned over easily and that I was limping, and then I asked which doctor she would suggest for me to talk to. I purposefully avoided the story about my leg feeling heavy. I wasn't ready for a psychiatrist yet! I ended up making an appointment with a foot doctor. With my collection of symptoms, he sounded as reasonable as anyone to me!

With my doctor appointment confirmed and our shopping done, we now returned home to our motel. It was there that we all agreed on a new venture for our group. To save on finances, we decided to do a little home cooking in our motel rooms. So, following our new decision it was back to the store for us. At least I had something to keep my mind on. I just limped along... angry.

After buying the basic essential items-coffee pot, skillet, and spatula-we were in business. We picked up our favorite boxed instant one pan skillet meal at the grocery store, plus a few other staples like a loaf of bread and some eggs for breakfast, and then went back to the motel to eat.

It was apparent from the start, which one of our group was the real cook. There was no contest. There was no competition for Frank.

Jerry and I were in charge of the silverware duty. This involved collecting utensils left on the meal trays, outside the other rooms, before room service had picked them up. It was a competitive duty requiring both agility and good timing. We confiscated, or rather borrowed, sugar, salt and pepper packages, cream containers and silverware. Then Jerry and I were also in charge of the after-meal clean up duty, which included hiding our borrowed collection.

Dinner went well. With Frank's cooking ability and Jerry and my teamwork, the meal was a tasty meal-saving success. After some self-rewarding praise, I was somehow elected to make breakfast the following day. This day will stand out in my mind for the rest of my life.

It all began with me making the coffee. Now, anyone should be able to make coffee... especially when someone else tells you how much coffee to put in the pot and how much water to add. These are generally the main ingredients.

I had my electric skillet warming up and my bag of frozen hash brown potatoes ready to go. At least the potatoes used to be frozen. Anyway, they were still cold from their place in the styrofoam ice chest, which we bought for our supplies.

There I was, me, in charge of breakfast. Cooking was not one of the skills I had mastered, or was interested in. This was my first chance to astound my partners. And that I did! I noticed a funny odor in my kitchen area and asked Frank if he smelled anything. He did and we were both going around the room from the window, to see if it was outside, to the skillet, trying to search out the origin of the odor. Jerry hadn't arrived yet to add his nose to the search.

Well, Frank finally found the problem. The coffee pot was up against the wall…or what used to be the wall… It had burned through the wallpaper and then through a portion of the wall itself. Once we got the fire out, we checked the coffee pot to discover that I had forgotten the water entirely and succeeded in burning out the electrical unit of our coffee maker. Ah, I'm such a cook… I've just never decided what kind. I just wanted to crawl into a hole and hide somewhere. Frank suggested that I forget the whole idea and suggested that I get a pot of coffee from the restaurant instead. My cooking must have scared him. He even volunteered to make breakfast.

I left for the restaurant, appreciating any kind of temporary escape. I was upset, but seemed to be coping with the situation all right. I ordered the coffee and sat down to wait while they brewed a new pot. When it was ready, they brought it out on a tray… in a glass container.

The glass was the first thing I saw. What a time to get fancy! Realizing that I was slightly limping, I knew that I'd have to really concentrate to get the coffee back to Frank's room, still in the glass pot. A guy from room service offered to carry it upstairs for me warning that the tray was heavy. Being a women's libber, I defiantly excused the warning. I'd waited for it, and I was right there, and I felt that I could handle it!

By now the coffee pot was becoming a personal challenge to me. I'd just have to walk slowly… The bell boy asked again if he could take it for me, which only made more determined to do it myself.

I slowly started back to Frank's room, concentrating on each step. I carefully limped down a hall, up the stairs and then down still another hall. I finally got to his door, still holding the tray, and carefully gave a slight foot knock. He opened the door.

The next thing I knew, the fancy glass pitcher slid across the tray and was on the floor and me. In typical female response, I started crying.

Upset, angry, and discouraged, I began picking up glass, looking through my tears. What was wrong with me! Frank was afraid I was going to cut myself on the glass. I was beyond caring at that point. He told me not to worry about it. I started for my room to cry some more before drying off.

After I'd straightened out a bit with the help of a little makeup, I returned to Frank's room to at least make an appearance at breakfast. Frank opened the door, but this time he jumped back holding up his hands to protect himself from whatever bad luck I had brought with me. I just smiled as a couple of new tears formed. But this time I was a little more in control of my emotions. I thanked Frank for cooking breakfast and explained that I had not only lost two coffee pots that morning, but I had also lost my appetite. But Jerry and he insisted that I eat something. Obstinately, I smoked a cigarette instead.

I then noticed that even it felt funny in my hand. But, I was still nervous and anything could have felt strange at that point. I still couldn't figure out how I had dropped the coffee. It happened so quickly. It just slid off the tray…

I still wasn't hungry that evening when Frank called suggesting that we go out to eat dinner. I was still worried about my leg; Frank was worried when I wasn't hungry. For the last few days I just hadn't been interested in eating. Since I had been known to "handle a mean knife and fork", I wouldn't consider myself a light eater. Any lack of appetite was always welcomed by me. I was pleased. I'd already lost about eight pounds!

But after a persistent effort by Frank, I finally gave in and agreed to go with him to eat at a little restaurant, which was close by. I don't recall the conversation on the way over, but I do remember Frank saying that since my leg was bothering me, we could stop at a hospital that was close and find out what exactly was wrong. I was concerned and agreed that we should stop, if I still had enough time to get ready for the show that evening. The night before I'd had some trouble rolling my hair and I wanted to make sure that I had plenty of time that night.

The next thing that I knew, we were pulling into the driveway at the "Emergency" entrance of a hospital. Nothing like quick service! When I signed in at the desk, I seemed to be having trouble writing my name. But for some reason, I just wasn't concerned about it at the time.

I had also been having some trouble playing the bass lately. Sometimes I'd hit the wrong string with my right hand. My left hand would be positioned on the correct note, but then I'd hit the wrong string with my right hand. Even playing my guitar seemed sloppier than my usual style. But nothing seemed to be adding up to make any sense. I had a number of unrelated strange problems, which weren't even constantly occurring.

After a short wait, my name was called and I was directed to an examination bed with the surrounding curtains pulled. I was then presented with a sheet and asked to disrobe. I wasn't quite sure what this all had to do with a leg problem, but I was open for any suggestions. Meanwhile, the lady on the other side of my curtain sounded like she was dying. This didn't give me any confidence.

After a while, my lady friend either quieted down or died, and my doctor came in and introduced himself. He asked a few initial questions and then let me do most of the talking, explaining my leg condition.

My examination was short. He did the usual "hammer on the knees" to test my reflexes, and ran something kind of sharp across the bottom of each of my feet. Then, he looked in my eyes, and felt my leg and ankle. Next, I was asked to sit up, close my eyes, with arms outstretched to my sides, and bring my two forefingers together to meet in front of me, keeping my arms straight. Then, holding my arms out straight with eyes still closed, I was supposed to touch my nose with each forefinger, first with one hand, then the other. Next, he touched me with the sharp or dull end of a pencil-like utensil. This little game went on with him touching different places on my forehead, face, and arms. He seemed to really get into this 'eyes closed' business!

The main test I recall from this brief examination was the number game. With eyes still closed, the doctor drew a number between one and ten in the palm of my hand, and asked me to identify it. I remember this because I felt that it was the one test which I failed. The numbers were all one digit, but once I got past the number one, I was confused. I couldn't figure out what he was writing. It didn't bother me though. I never did well in math...

My total examination lasted about five minutes. I was then asked to get dressed and to meet my doctor in his office. This whole thing seemed kind of silly. He had done so little that I didn't know how he expected to find anything out. I expected to hear the old, "according to my tests, you seem to be fine" routine. How could anyone diagnose a leg problem from a few-wrong numbers?

I went into his office and closed the door behind me. Being on Emergency duty, he didn't waste any time. He felt that there was something definitely wrong with me. I was relieved to find that at least we agreed.

He then told me that he believed that my problem was in the brain. He continued to say that certain messages were not being transmitted properly. He suggested that I go into the hospital in Olympia. His alternative choice was for me to fly home immediately, get a good neurosurgeon, and go directly into a hospital in Colorado.

Now this was a surprise! I never knew that numbers were that important! My Olympia entertainment contract ran through the following weekend and then continued for another full week. I immediately wondered what Frank and Jerry's reaction would be to my news...

To add a little credibility to my story, I asked the doctor if he would repeat his Medical suggestions to my partner. He agreed to, and I called Frank into his office. He then repeated his diagnosis while praising the qualified neurologists and neurosurgeons who were available at the hospital there.

He must have made an impression on Frank. He was concerned. I seemed to be the only one who was concerned about the booking! But I now had a chance to go home, and I decided to take it. The doctor asked me to stop at his hospital on my way to the airport to pick up a report of his diagnosis. We agreed to, and left.

I still couldn't believe it! My hospital stop turned into a one-way ticket home! At least he had recognized that something was wrong with me. A leg examination pointed to my brain. I guess it was all in my head after all!

Before we left, he told me that my problem could be anything from a minor nervous disorder to Multiple Sclerosis. Since I wasn't familiar with either, I thought I'd just go home and get a few more opinions from the Colorado medical world.

I left the hospital in good spirits, joking with Frank about my problem being in the brain. I had nothing to lose there! Now that my problem had been identified, I was even getting hungry. Once we were back at the car, I asked Frank where that restaurant of his was. But I was too late... Apparently while I was playing number games with the doctor, Frank had eaten in the cafeteria at the hospital.

So for me, it was a hamburger and a chocolate shake at the closest drive-in, but it tasted better than ever... I was going home!

We soon arrived back at the motel and explained my new surprise diagnosis to Jerry. My next step was to contact a neurosurgeon. I was totally lost in my approach to this. Thankfully, Frank and Jerry took over for me. I packed, preparing for my trip, while Frank called a friend of his, a doctor in Fort Collins, who referred him to a capable neurosurgeon in Denver. Meanwhile, Jerry checked plane schedules and made reservations for me.

With suitcases full, I returned to Frank's room to receive my new doctor's name and phone number. I then called him, only to find out that he would be out of town for the coming weekend, leaving early the next morning. Since it was Friday and my flight didn't arrive in Denver until after midnight, it appeared that I would miss my new specialist. He certainly didn't sound over-anxious to see me. But I was feeling very agreeable and decided to go into the hospital in Denver and just wait to see him on Monday. He did offer me a number to call if I needed him before he returned, but, when I attempted to write it down, I found that I couldn't control my pen at all. The number was unintelligible. I still wasn't overly concerned, just frustrated, as I asked Frank to take the number for me.

Obviously concerned, Frank then took the phone and got not only the number, but a commitment from the doctor to meet me at the hospital the next morning at 4 a.m., before leaving on his business trip. In 15 seconds, Frank had achieved what I had been unable to do in several minutes. I was thankful and relieved. It's always nice to know that your doctor will be there, if you need him...

I didn't seem to be thinking very straight. Everything was happening so quickly... My condition seemed to be worsening. Frank realized that time was very important in halting the progression of a disease. A friend of ours had lost his hearing due to this mistake. It could possibly have been saved if his problem had been identified earlier.

I was obviously confused and incapable of organizing my new hospital move, so I tried to just relax while Frank and Jerry handled the situation for me.

I still needed to call my husband, Bob. All of this excitement in Olympia, and he was unaware, sleeping in Denver. I woke him up. I told him that I was coming home and asked him to pick me up at the airport at 3 a.m. I then further explained that I wasn't actually coming home, but that I needed to go directly to the hospital. I briefly told him that I was limping, something was wrong with my leg, and I was going into the hospital for further tests. I suggested that he sleep a couple of hours more and said that I'd see him soon.

I guess he didn't go back to sleep... He called Frank back in a few minutes, this time fully awake, to verify his dream and to find out what was actually happening...

But it wasn't a dream... it was real... and no one knew what was happening...

# ***FLY HIGH***

*I'm gonna fly high on a big bird,*
*In the middle of some very dark night.*
*And trace a distant pattern down below,*
*Through the maze of multi-colored lights.*

*I'm gonna fly high on a big bird,*
*Look down on a million living dots below.*
*And ask myself why other worlds appear so small,*
*Looking out through my reflection in the window.*

> *No smoking . . . fasten seatbelts . . .*
> *All seats upright . . .*
> *There's a stereo program provided just for you,*
> *Hope you have a very nice flight.*

> *This is you captain . . . the stewardess will serve you . . .*
> *Soft drinks or alcohol instead.*
> *If the cabin pressurizer should begin to fail,*
> *An O2 mask will fall upon your head.*

*(sing verses together)*
*I'm gonna fly high . . . . (repeat, fade)*

After a brief stop to pick up my Olympia report, I was on my way to the airport. I checked in at the reservation desk while Frank quietly ordered a wheelchair for me. I wanted to walk, or limp, down the concourse, but both Frank and Jerry insisted that I should ride in the chair. Outnumbered, I finally gave in and sat down.

Only then did I realize how self-conscious I felt about riding in a wheelchair. It seemed to me that I was causing a commotion, making a scene at the airport. I guess the only commotion was within myself...

I remember being very aware of the fact that I was on a different physical level than everyone. I was below them... I was always looking up at other people, feeling inferior, and very conspicuous. I preferred looking down at people from the stage.

Aside from my wheelchair complex, I felt quite normal. The emotional mood of our group was light and cheerful. Sincere concern was hidden with nervous laughter. The wheelchair became a new toy for us, a possible escape for any tension, which developed. We smoked... and joked... and waited for my plane...

When my departure time arrived, I said my thank-yous and good-byes, while assuring everyone that I'd be fine travelling alone. I was tough. I didn't need anyone's support. Then, I was wheeled over to the ramp leading onto the plane. The attendant asked me if I could walk, and I responded with an unconcerned, "sure..." Then he helped me as I limped on to the plane.

I had an aisle seat. I think they isolated me purposefully. No one sat beside me. But, I was satisfied since this was the first chance I'd had to relax since I had decided to go to dinner with Frank the night before. So I sat back, put on my earphones, and checked the musical program which was being offered.

Relaxing with the music, I watched the lights on the ground as we left Olympia. As I looked out, the lights inside of the plane made a reflection of my face in the window. It reminded me of a song, which I had written: "I'm gonna fly high on a big bird/in the middle of some very dark night/and trace a distant pattern down below/through the maze of multicolored lights. I'm gonna fly high on a bird/look down on a million living dots below/and ask myself why other worlds appear so small/looking out through my reflection in the window."

It always amazes me to realize that all of those tiny lights represent many different people, whose personal lives, problems, decisions, and dreams are equally as important to them as mine are to me.

My light watching was finally interrupted by the stewardess taking drink orders from the passengers. I couldn't pass up taking advantage of the free coke and peanuts, which were offered.

The peanuts not only tasted good, but they also revealed a new problem to me. While putting a peanut in my mouth, my fingers had accidentally touched my lips. My lips were now numb... I quickly felt my face and found that my entire right cheek seemed numb.

I thought that maybe I was still imagining these things... So much had happened in such a short period of time that I felt capable of imagining just about anything. I had purposely avoided concentrating on the reason for my trip. I didn't wish to dwell on the problems, which had been occurring to me. I couldn't seem to figure out what was wrong... so I had stopped trying. Now I chose to ignore my numbness discovery and concentrate on the music, which was playing. I can lose myself in music until that's all I can hear or think about. Thankfully, I got lost that night...

I moved over to my window seat before we began our descent into Denver. I wanted to see all of those lights again.

I was anxious to see my husband after having been gone for three weeks. Sitting near the back of the plane, I knew I wouldn't be one of the first people off. But, as soon as I limped through the plane and down the enclosed ramp, Bob was there. What a welcome sight! He felt great, but the guy with the wheelchair standing beside him didn't look quite as welcoming to me. Apparently Frank had ordered the wheelchair to be available upon my arrival while Bob had asked for the electrical baggage cart to be there. The cart appeared much more impressive to me. We dismissed the wheelchair.

I got in with my suitcase, rode past the airline gates, and into the main terminal. And after riding in each, I can only say, electrical carts sure beat wheelchairs for travelling...

Now, it was back to the hospital for me. Not the same hospital that I had been in seven hours before in Olympia, but a new Colorado hospital, Rose Memorial Hospital. If you've seen one hospital, you've generally seen them all…. But, there were some differences. There was no rain here, and I was home. The Colorado air was fresh and clean. It was a beautiful night. I was safe and secure and my husband was with me…

We got to the hospital where I scribbled in, while they called my doctor for me. He was at home; trying to sleep as much as possible before his business weekend began. He must have lived near the hospital; it wasn't long before he arrived.

Meanwhile, I was issued my hospital gown and bracelet, neither of which I really wanted. But, I was concerned about my condition and interested in identifying my problem.

Naturally, I was anxious to begin some kind of medication or treatment for my improvement. Something was wrong with me, and I wanted to know what it was, what I could expect, and what could be done for me. Now I was only interested in answers.

Soon my long distance neurologist came into my waiting room introducing himself as Dr. Stanley Ginsburg. The examination, which followed, seemed to be a repeat of my emergency physicians in Olympia, with a few added specialties. Again, the tests seemed so simple that I didn't understand how anyone could determine anything.

This doctor did seem more interested in the way in which I was limping. He asked me to walk toward him and then away from him several times. Then, laying on my back, I was asked to hold each leg straight up, one at a time, while the doctor would push it back down to the table. I thought that he was checking my muscles at that point. (Legs are one of my best attributes…)

I explained what had occurred to me while I was in Olympia and expressed my concern about the rapid progression of my problems. By now, the entire right side of my face was numb, something which had occurred since my last hospital examination only a few hours before.

Dr. Ginsburg was sincere and frank while trying not to be overly alarming. He told me, if I had what he thought it was, I might not regain the full use of my right hand.... He continued to say that with the medication he was prescribing, my right leg should improve significantly. I would be entering the hospital for further tests, in order to make a definite determination of my problem. He would see me when he returned on Monday...

I wanted answers. I had gotten them... At least, enough for one night.

I couldn't sleep. I had been awake for almost twenty-one hours and now I was exhausted. But I couldn't sleep. I couldn't escape the reality of my problem, the possisbility of having a lifetime physical disability. Now I was less interested in a diagnosis and more inerested in a treatment. Anything, which could destroy the use of my hand, was serious. And any medication, which could allow me to walk normally again, seemed miraculous.

It was quite a change for me, coming from Olympia, Washington, to Rose Memorial Hospital. The night before, I had been in my Olympian motel, anxious to go on stage, and now I was in a Colorado hospital, anxious to regain yesterday's normality. The states were different, there was a time difference, and my purpose for being in each place was very different. The only thing, which both places did have in common, was changing the bed sheets every night.

But at least I would get a good rest. At least, I thought I would... After being there for two weeks, I realized that people who intend to rest in a hospital are either those who've never been in one before, or those who can afford the quiet of a private room. I was the first type who soon discovered that nothing is free. You have to pay for rest...

Since I hadn't planned this trip, or made any reservations ahead of time, I had a roommate. At least I thought I did... The curtain between our beds was drawn. My arrival didn't seem to affect my friend's sleep. The snoring continued uninterrupted.

I didn't sleep at all on that first night. I just laid in bed, wondering, and watching the room get lighter with the sun.

Finally, some commotion in the hall suggested that my first

hospital day was officially beginning. The nurse came in. Apparently it was blood pressure and temperature check time. Unknowingly, this would become a very routine procedure for me. Window curtains were then opened and morning was rudely announced by the sun. At this point, I was beginning to wonder if I had mistakenly enlisted in the army instead of a hospital.

I wasn't in my most pleasant mood since I hadn't slept, but this sunrise wake up service was totally off my schedule. This was the first time I'd been up this early in years! Or, at least this was the first time I had been awakened this early. The life of an entertainer is not a normal 8 to 5-work shift. I usually performed from 9 at night until 2 the next morning. Then it was not unusual for me to go out for breakfast with friends and drink about a gallon of coffee as major decisions and problems in life were being solved. Generally, my being up at sunrise was interpreted as a suggestion that it was time for me to go to bed, not to get up.

But the hospital had different ideas. Breakfast came shortly after the grand opening of the curtains. Again, this was different. I usually ate breakfast at 3 or 4 a.m., after work, or at noon, when I finally did get up. It seemed that these people were always either too early, or too late for me.

They were also pretty nosy. They asked me if I had to go to the bathroom. I couldn't believe it! I could still walk! What did going to the bathroom have to do with a minor hand or leg problem? I assured them that I was quite comfortable at the time. I was then told to turn my light on, to call for the nurse, when I did need to go. Evidently, I wasn't supposed to get up by myself. Now, I was even restricted to my bed.

It sounded like my roommate was either a female, or a guy with a very high voice. I wasn't familiar with hospital regulations. Whoever it was, they weren't interested in breakfast and preferred sleeping. I agreed. At least we had something in common. She was either sleeping, or snored while she was awake.

After breakfast came the bedding change. My nurse reappeared to ask if I was ready for my bath. She didn't ask if I would care to take a bath, but rather if I was ready to take it. I was getting closer and closer to a dishonorable discharge from this army-style enlistment.

My bath water was run for me, and I was helped into the bathroom, and then even into the tub. I must admit that I was glad that the nurse was there for the tub part. With my leg, it was a bit of a problem. But, someone else should have run the bath water. It was only lukewarm. Now I'm not sure what temperature lukewarm is, but I know this water should have been hotter.

The nurse washed my back and told me to wait for her to return before getting out. As soon as she left, I turned the hot water on and mixed it around some. I then washed, and waited. I waited, and waited, and waited…

Soon I decided to make a little noise to remind someone of my waterlogged condition. My nurse had checked on me once since I'd been in the tub, but it had been some time ago, before I was ready to get out. Now that I was ready, I seemed to be the only one. Not knowing her name, and not wishing to alarm anyone else, I tried to attract a little attention with a faint, "yoo hoo?" I don't know where I got that idea, but it seemed to be appropriate at the time. I only tried it twice. It sounded so ridiculous to me that I finally decided to relax and wait patiently. Shortly after, the nurse arrived to rescue me. By now, I felt as wrinkled as a prune, but I was clean!

Now I could sleep, or I would have been able to sleep, if they had only let me. Each time that I was awakened, I disliked it more, and more. "Their" lunch, and patient check schedule, came right in the middle of "my" night…

Even when "their" night came, I still had interruptions. Both my husband and my parents arrived, anxious to inspect my condition. Everyone asked the same question, "What's wrong?" That's why I was there, to be tested and to find out.

As my hospital stay continued, Bob did something which was very important for me. He called our friends, telling them where I was, and encouraging them to call me, to keep my spirits up. Looking back, I can now appreciate my husband's forethought and realize the importance of receiving those calls. Between the hospital routine and the telephone, I didn't have time to worry!

The next day, I began physical therapy (P.T.). This means

that I went to the therapy room, which specialized in external or physical treatment of the body for disabilities, injuries, or diseases. This immediate transition from the lifestyle of an entertainer to the awareness of handicapped and crippled people was a mental shock in itself for me. I had never known anyone who was disabled, and I certainly didn't consider myself in that category. But there I was, in my hospital wheelchair, being rolled into a room offering therapy for adjustment into society. There I was, generally the star of the show, now merely a role player in a production of misfortunate characters.

I felt very strange and very uneasy. Those of us who are fortunate enough to have good health are not familiar with abnormalities. It seems we fear the unusual, the unknown. And somehow, those who are afflicted must recognize this uneasiness of others and then quietly avoid these personal associations.

Children generally react to disabilities cruelly. The visible difference seems first to be inquisitively observed and then regarded humorously. Teasing and laughing act as an emotional release, a substitute for the lack of understanding. An adult reaction may be displayed differently, but it still can be just as cruel. P.T. patients are just beginning a transition period. Physical aids can be provided and their operation learned, but the psychological adjustment is dependent on the patient.

I learned one thing from this room beyond my exercises and skill games. I gained a great respect for physical therapists. They are the people whose job is encouraging others, to help themselves.

The therapist ends up being a psychiatrist, exercise leader, and morale booster, all in one. Often their help is needed before it is desired. The patient may be trying to adjust to the loss of a limb or to a disease, while exercise is still necessary to retain the use of their uninjured muscles. At least, this is my understanding. And I, as others who I witnessed, was not in the least interested in "adjustment" or "rehabilitation."

My respect for physical therapists was not gained immediately. In fact, I learned to hate my twice-a-day visit to therapy. The therapists would talk a great deal, ask questions, and encourage me to respond. They seemed to be too nice. I resented their happy, smiling faces, and exuberant approach toward activities. It just didn't seem genuine. It seemed more like a game, a game that I didn't want to play.

There was one patient in P.T. who I particularly did enjoy. She was suffering from the pain of crippling arthritis in her hands. She seemed as disenchanted with her therapy visits as I did.

One time the therapist enthusiastically suggested to my friend, "How would you like to sew today?" Her mistake was making it a question. The patient calmly responded, "I don't want to sew." The therapist now approached it from a new angle, something more timely, suggesting that they create a Christmas stocking as a gift. My friend repeated, "I don't want to sew." The therapist reminded the patient that the doctor wanted to see her work and it was necessary to work on skills that were lost if she wanted to ever regain them. The answer remained the same, "I don't want to sew." In her final effort, the therapist threatened that the doctor would be notified. My friend repeated her same rejection more emphatically this time.

Quietly listening on the outside, I was inwardly cheering support for her refusal. I wondered to myself, now what would they do? What could they do? Although the patient never sewed, I'm not really sure who won...

Since I had arrived at the hospital, my lameness had worsened in a matter of days. I was now unable to move either my right foot or my right toes at all. My writing problem had digressed to a total lack of coordination on my right side: hand, fingers, and arm.

I went to P.T. twice a day, twenty minutes each time, in two separate rooms. One area was for exercising my leg and helping me to walk, while the other concentrated on my arm and hand.

To me, this daily exercise routine seemed like a waste of time. It always interrupted my nap time. I wasn't having any trouble sleeping these days, although I couldn't blame that on the therapy. It wasn't that strenuous. No one asked me to sew, but I was coerced into typing. I hadn't typed for years, but I had learned at one time. Now, typing was considered good exercise for my fingers. I had been having some vision difficulties lately, so large print was required for my copying exercise.

I was not particularly opposed to typing, until I tried. It must have been a long time since I had typed... I was terrible! First of all, I had trouble reading the print which I was to copy. Second, my fingers didn't go where I wanted them to, third my right hand kept falling down an entire row on the keys, and last, the concentrated effort gave me a headache each day. If my friend didn't like sewing, she should have tried typing! Following her example, I told my leaders that I didn't want to type. Avoiding a battle, we settled on a compromise. I got away with less time at the typewriter.

"Theraplast," a substance like silly putty, was used for strengthening my fingers and hand. I had different finger exercises, pulling against the putty's resistance. Then, I was taught how to perform such simple tasks as buttoning my robe and just getting it on and off, somehow. It sounds easy enough, but I just couldn't make my hand do what I wanted it to. And, there were block games. One had wooden pieces that looked like empty spools of thread. The object of this game was to put the pieces into indentures in a block of wood. There were no decisions, or strategies in this game, just moving the spools from one place to another, where they would fit. This would have been a simple enough task under normal conditions. But, my right arm and hand, seemed to have a mind of their own. They would dart off in the direction of their choice.

I can't begin to describe the frustration I experienced. I wasn't accomplishing what I had intended. No one likes to be defeated... I never was a good loser...especially when I was being defeated by simple maneuvers, which I had always taken for granted.

I even had trouble eating. Often I'd become frustrated with the silverware, and would revert to eating with my fingers. I never imagined that I would experience the spastic-like movements which were now present in my arm and in my hand.

My right leg also had some noticeable lack of control. This was visible in my exercising. It not only felt heavy, but the muscles also seemed very weak.

As if this weren't enough, I next began having problems with my equilibrium. After my exercises, I would try to walk a little, either holding on to my assistant, or being aided by crutches. Eventually, I graduated to a cane.

I didn't feel very stable with any of these, and finally decided that they were doing this therapy entirely wrong. How could I walk, when I felt like I was going to fall? And if I did begin to fall, how could I catch myself with a cane? I wasn't even sure of which direction to push, to prevent a fall...

It seemed utterly ridiculous to me to be concerned with walking, when just standing made me dizzy. First things must come first! I decided that when my head cleared up, then I would work on my walking. It never occurred to me that the dizziness and motion might never go away...

My morale seemed good, overall. My husband and my brother deserve most of the credit for morale boosting. Whatever fears they may have had about my health were well masked with their sarcasm and teasing. Like two little boys, their antics kept me smiling. Like men, their concern was hidden, their encouragement emphasized.

I had been taking two shots a day of some kind of cortisone stimulant called "ACTH" as my treatment. I thought it seemed to be helping, but my condition still fluctuated so. It definitely helped my foot. I could now move it again. I could even bend my toes! That was my first sign in the right direction. Then, the numbness in my face gradually faded away...

I didn't mind the shots. I just wanted more of this miracle drug.

The doctor said it should also help my vision. Both of my eyes were now terrible. It's difficult to describe what I did see. It seemed like something was in my eyes, but I couldn't feel anything. Everything appeared as if it were behind a cloudy, or foggy, window which was smudged with dirt which blocked my vision. There was no secretion, but I thought that it must be a mucous substance inside my eyes because it seemed to move.

My eyes also seemed as uncoordinated as the entire right side of my body. They didn't focus together. It seemed like I was looking through someone else's glasses, someone with very poor eyesight. My eyes felt very strained. So most of my days, for the first week and a half, were spent sleeping, or resting, with my eyes closed. I couldn't read, or watch TV. I couldn't even sign Christmas cards for my friends.

Everything seemed so variable. I'd wake up some mornings, and things would look more normal to me. I'd think that I could see better, and believe that the shots were finally working. Then, the next morning I'd wake up, and my eyesight would seem worse again. It was so changeable, and so discouraging. It seemed like I was taking two steps forward, and then three steps backwards.

I complained to the doctor about my daily headaches after therapy. The ride down to P.T. even bothered me. The motion of the wheelchair seemed exaggerated. That, plus the strain on my eyes, made the trip totally unbearable. Sometimes I even felt faint, and nauseated, by the time I got down there. Dr. Ginsburg suggested that I close my eyes and try that. It seemed to work better. My headaches even seemed fewer.

When I wasn't sleeping, I was taking my temperature, or blood pressure, eating, talking on the phone, visiting with my parents, relatives, and friends, going down for a test, or providing urine samples. Getting one sample was a trick in itself. The hospital provides you with your own personal sterilized kit. The instruction sheet, for step by step procedure, could be printed as a book. For those who are unfamiliar with this procedure, may I suggest starting early, before you need to go… The instruction material is lengthy, and explicit, and doesn't allow time for slow readers or confusion. When the doctor wants a sample, he wants it now! Even if you haven't had a drink in a week…

Friends are the people everyone needs… I felt very fortunate. I never realized how important phone calls and visitors could be, until I was in the hospital. My room began to look like a greenhouse! I received so many beautiful plants and flowers. I never did well with plants. I couldn't tell one flower from another, but they were all colorful. But, the more I received, the more I began to wonder about my friends' intentions. I always thought you sent flowers when someone died…

By this time, I had a new roommate. I never got to be close friends with the old one. No time for empathy. I guess we both were too concerned with our own personal problems.

My new roommate had come for heart surgery, generally recognized as a valve job. She was a wonderful, and enlightening woman. I left the hospital the day she was supposed to be operated on. I prayed for her...

She took care of my flowers and me, in typical motherly style. Being from out of Denver, a three-hour drive in good weather, her husband and son were unable to visit her often. She did have a sister, living within bus distance, who got over whenever possible.

I felt badly... I had so many friends and relatives who visited and sent me flowers. Life seems so unfair at times. She placed my flowers and planters on the ledge by the window, and watered them daily. Even the plants knew they were loved...

There's a test for everything in the hospital. I was about to begin my first testing era. Combined with my fear of hospitals, each new test became a slight trauma for me. I was still in no pain, and I wasn't anxious to begin to be. During my three weeks in the hospital, I believe I was tested for everything testable.

It all began with a direction from the doctors; "No more birth control pills." You can imagine how thrilled I was with this decision since I'd been away from my husband for three and a half weeks. But I consented. There's not that many intimate opportunities in a hospital.

Their next order was; "Don't get pregnant." Sure... They took away my pills, and then said don't get pregnant, all in the same breath. Then they sent me to a gynecologist at the hospital to receive more information on new, improved methods of birth control. I wondered if this would help my right side...

In my new vulnerable condition, my husband decided that a little male nudity might liven up my hospital stay. He brought me a Playgirl magazine...the liberated woman's answer to Playboy. Men become the featured models of this publication. My new reading material made quite a hit with the nurses but, unfortunately, my poor eyesight prevented me from enjoying the detailed photographs.

The nurses weren't the only ones who were interested in my new magazine. Young interns also became curious. Since the doctors had taken so many pictures (x-rays) of me, I felt that it was only fair if I could take a few pictures of them. After suggesting the idea, I didn't get any offers… just smiles.

My testing era included x-rays of both my head and my body. I doubt that the head x-rays were very complicated. I'm sure they were checking for tumors. The possibility of a brain tumor had not been ruled out.

Then there was an accumulation of standard tests on my blood, kidneys, eyes, bones, and bladder, plus a few specimens, an EEG examination, and a spinal tap.

From my limited understanding, the EEG, the electroencephalogram, is supposed to measure electrical brain waves. I assume the patterns of thought are represented on a graph. Although I have no idea what is determined, or how, I can explain the patient's perspective.

Some type of cold liquid was spotted all over my head. I imagine this either acts as some type of a conductor to register the electrical impulses, or as a glue for the rubber-like suction cups, which were then stuck onto my head. Each little cup had a wire attached to it, which was then attached to the graph apparatus. I didn't have a mirror, but I assume that I ended up looking like a dropout from a UFO, an Unidentified Flying Object, a dropout with little suction cups and wires coming out of my head. I was a bit skeptical about this procedure, but I remained unharmed.

I'm not sure how long this test lasted. There was quiet music playing in the office while I was getting "stuck up," and I ended up dozing off to sleep. Possibly, they may have stimulated one particular area to induce the sleep. I have no idea if that's even possible. But, it was rather embarrassing to find out that I'd slept through the entire procedure.

In another test they injected a special fluid into the vein of my right arm and then watched the liquid circulate through my body on a type of x-ray television. They were checking for blockages again, I assume.

Then there were the kidney and bladder x-rays, one of which was done in the surgical room of the hospital.

Eye examinations were done on a machine with lights and a buzzer. Focusing on a central point, I was supposed to push the buzzer button when I first saw any moving light. A varying sized dot traveled into view from different directions. For me, this test also was a tiring procedure. I knew I did poorly when an aid took me back for more tests the next day, and remarked about how tired I must have been the previous day.

My big test was the spinal tap. I was told that a fluid would be injected at the base of my spine and would be watched, like the others, to check again for any blockage. I would be strapped to a movable table top with a camera overhead which transmitted the flow of the liquid to a TV set screen in the same room. The idea was to tilt the table until I felt like I'd fall on my head, and then, tilt it back until I was almost standing erect. I was able to watch the TV. After entertaining for years, I'd always wanted to be on television. But this wasn't exactly what I'd had in mind.

The one thing that the doctors avoided telling me, which I soon discovered, was that the fluid, that was injected, may cause nausea. But thankfully, it was only temporary, and there still was no pain.

The major concern with this test was the possibility of headaches following the spinal. I was to remain horizontal for several hours. I was told not to sit up at all. With all of the headaches I'd been experiencing lately, I certainly wasn't interested in any new types. I think they must have given me a sedative in my preparation shots. It helped me to stay down. I sure slept well.

I emerged from my testing era with a new respect for doctors. Each of mine had taken time to explain what was being done to me, and what I could expect to occur. Their open and frank approach resulted in my believing in them, and my dependency on their decisions.

I've heard of patients falling in love with their doctors. Now I can realize why this feeling might occur. I was so dependent on my doctor's decisions. My life was beyond my control. I can now understand that this feeling, of totally needing another individual, could mistakenly be interpreted as love. Basic desires for survival become very evident in a hospital situation.

I seemed to be improving. I'd been in the hospital for three weeks. I only knew that I was ready to go home. But I hadn't heard anything from the doctors. They still came by every day with their questions, and asked me to do their simple coordination tests. I was even the subject of inspection for a class, a group of young interns. The interns asked me everything from identifying a writing pen to a memory test of repeating several sentences in a row. With that group of doctors, I didn't mind being the subject of inspection. I'm still an entertainer at heart...

Still, nothing had been said to me. What was wrong? As long as they continued testing, I didn't expect an answer. By now, I was beginning to feel less anxious. Maybe I didn't want to know. Anyway I wasn't particularly interested in the medical terminology identifying my problem.

I already knew that my right arm and leg weren't operating properly. But, I guess I still wanted someone to tell me what was wrong. At least, I felt like once it was diagnosed, it could be treated. Had my rodeo and horse injuries finally caught up with me? Could an injury cause a disease?

Dr. Ginsburg came by every day, or sent his associates by when he was out of town. At least I was popular. I did know that I'd lost about fifteen pounds, which I was proud of. (I mean I was proud of losing them.) I think all women are proud to lose weight. Thinness is in!

I was discouraged with a portion of my weight loss. I think it came mostly from my chest. There wasn't much there to begin with, but now there seemed to be even less.

I also made a new discovery about my face. I could die of starvation, and my face would still look fat. I've always had a round face, a type of cherub look, and I've always envied women with those thin faces and striking cheekbones. There just seems to be something about women whose cheeks look withdrawn that adds some mysterious appeal. (Starvation) But now, I realized that my round face wasn't necessarily due to my weight. So, I guess my face will always be round, and I will continue to be envious.

Overall, my condition seemed to be worse than when I'd come into the hospital, three weeks before, but better than I had experienced, at my lowest point, while in the hospital. So, I seemed to be getting better. My coordination in both my arms and legs seemed to be improving. The numbness in my face would still come, and go. My headaches were still occurring, but not as severely as they had been. I still wasn't allowed to get out of bed alone, not even to go to the bathroom. In fact they had started putting up the side rails on my bed each night. I wasn't sure if they expected me to escape, but I appreciated any suggestion of that possibility. At least I felt secure.

The doctors always asked me if I was experiencing any sensations of motion. I wasn't. But I suspected this to be the reason for the bars.

I had noticed some unusual feelings, when I was in the bathtub, though I blamed this on my eyes. The movement of the water seemed exaggerated. Each bath for me seemed to be a miniature ocean storm with waves crashing in on me, like the Titanic, from all sides. Luckily, I never got seasick.

P.T. was still a bummer. Challenging, yes, but somehow I seemed destined to lose. I was making some progress in the arm and hand department, but walking was a much different story. In fact it was just ridiculous! I was visibly off balance... I just had to hold on to someone.

They first started me with a type of short crutches with a metal arm brace (Canadian Crutches). I didn't do very well... I then tried regular crutches. The therapist apparently was more satisfied with these, but I still didn't do well. Finally, I ended up with a cane. It was suggested that I buy one of these, which could easily be billed to my hospital account. I did. I acquired my own personal piece of wood.

The lack of balance, which I was experiencing, made me appear to be intoxicated... drunk. But everyone knew that the hospital didn't offer those opportunities! Sex and alcohol were not choices.

Still someone in P.T. must have been wondering about me for my tests were geared accordingly. I was asked to walk along a white line. Now this was a joke to me. They had to be kidding! In my condition, I was lucky if I even saw the white line, to begin with. Even then, my balance was so poor that this was an impossible task.

I staggered forward a few steps to make an effort. From then on, my walking alone, unassisted, was done between two bars, where

I could catch myself from falling. I repeated my earlier suggestion, "As soon as my head gets straight, then I'll worry about walking."

But, now I had my cane. I never did figure out how I was supposed to catch myself with a cane, but they were determined that I practice walking with it. I was just glad that they were within catching distance so I wouldn't impale myself.

My entertainment partners called me almost daily from Olympia. They'd stayed in Washington to finish out the booking as a duo rather than our original trio. They assured me that there was no need to worry about the act.

I wasn't worried. I was beyond worrying. I just wanted to get my head straightened out. I knew they were interested and concerned. There was one question which affected each of us though. Would I be able to perform again?

Dr. Ginsburg's only immediate answer was that I could do anything that I felt like doing, but we'd just have to wait. He did suggest that I didn't change my entire lifestyle. I should just use a little discretion, and do things in moderation. My questions could only be answered by time.

So I told Frank and Jerry, we'd just have to wait. But waiting is the one thing that is the most difficult in a profession that is dependent on timely opportunities. And, waiting doesn't feed people. We had entertainment contracts for a couple of months in advance, but since the act was changed by "an act of God," the guys were not committed to perform. But, entertainers rely on the income which is contracted ahead of time.

Frank and Jerry's time in Olympia would be a definite turning point for our group. I think everyone tends to get naturally lazy, losing inspiration, until a need occurs and a decision has to be made. This case was a definite "have to" situation. There were bills to be paid, new moves to be made.

Each was achieved. Scheduled dates were cancelled and new directions initiated. Thankfully, I was never actually eliminated or even replaced.

Then early one morning, after our usual question and discussion period, Dr. Ginsburg sat down on my bed and looked at me very seriously. His diagnosis was ready.

He began his medical explanation by comparing my nerves to a telephone wire, referring to the insulation on the wires. He explained that the insulation around my nerves was inflamed. The inflamation was breaking the transmission of messages from my brain to certain areas of my body. He compared it to a link missing in a chain.

When he first began talking, I didn't understand the terminology he was using. I interrupted him, admitting my ignorance, and asked for a simple discription. He answered that I would recognize this condition as "Multiple Sclerosis." He paused, waiting for my reaction. This was the second time I'd heard of this disease. And it was still a mystery to me...I simply answered, "ok".

I was neither shocked nor astounded. My "ok" was just an acceptance. I didn't know a thing about Multiple Sclerosis. I never knew anyone who had it, and I didn't have any idea what to expect. But, regardless, it would have to be "OK." The doctors had arrived at a decision. It was not my choice. Rejection was meaningless.

After identifying my problem, my doctor's next sentence was a shock. "M.S. is not curable...but it is controllable." Now this was a surprise! I had an incurable disease? Me? I had a disease which could be with me for the rest of my life?

They had identified my problem, but there was no treatment for curing it! What always seems to happen to someone else, was now actually happening to me...

After accepting the fact that the disease was incurable, I was totally dependent on Dr. Ginsburg's last word, "controllable". If he said it was controllable, I was satisfied and relieved. Everything was still "OK".

I was told that if I felt like crying, hollering or whatever other release of emotions I needed, he would understand. He then explained that most people who have M.S. lead a near normal life. I was satisfied with that, never questioning his definitions of "near normal".

It took a while for my new information to sink in enough to be partially digested. When it did, the questions began in my mind. Was

M.S. hereditary? What caused it? But again, I wasn't overly anxious for the answers.

My first concern was about having children. I'd been singing professionally for years, never taking the time to have the children which both my husband and I desired. I was told that M.S. doesn't seem to be hereditary and women who had been diagnosed with the disease still had families. But there was a chance of having more problems during pregnancy than normally occur. Again, I was satisfied with the answer. Everything still seemed all right.

In fact, I was almost relieved by all of my recent answers. Entertainment can be a very demanding profession. You are constantly being judged by other people while trying to achieve your own personal goals. Stardom is the desired goal, but the definition of accomplishment varies according to the entertainer. I wonder if any entertainer is ever satisfied? Is there really some end to be achieved?

Our group had recorded two albums and we were scheduled to cut our third in January. I guess I would be considered a successful entertainer. I'd experienced life through other people, studying and entertaining them. I was doing something which I enjoyed, hoping that it was equally as enjoyable to my audience.

I'd like to think that I entertained solely to satisfy other people. But I'm afraid that wouldn't be entirely true. It's a very self satisfying experience for the entertainer. And egotistically, the applause feels good...

I had tried to determine why I was entertaining. My only decision was, that I enjoyed it. Booking, and promoting the act plus traveling and performing can be frustrating at times, but some unexplainable desire to perform pushed me onward.

Entertaining is addictive. Once you're into it, you're hooked. Withdrawal can be painful.

But now I was relieved. I believe it was because I'm such a poor loser. Now I had an excuse, a legitimate excuse for discontinuing my efforts. At times, I had felt so close to my goal of success, and yet I may have been very far away. I'd been enthusiastic, anxious, and discouraged so many times, experiencing the normal ups and downs of all entertainers. Someone once told me that entertainers experience more extremes of emotion than anyone else, the highest highs and the lowest lows. I think they must have been an entertainer.

Now I was somewhere in the middle. I didn't win, and I didn't lose. I'd simply been eliminated from the game. I had received an honorable discharge. I was eliminated and free to begin a family. Without my new excuse, it would have been difficult for me to just "drop out". Now it almost seemed as if I had been waiting for this to retire.


Doctor Ginsburg told me that I could stay in the hospital being tested forever, but if I would prefer, he was going to let me go home. I'm not really sure what he said after that. The only part I heard was, "I could go home."

Thinking back, he mentioned something about more tests, which could be done on the brain. This statement didn't actually register with me until the next day. Did he mean that this disease could affect my brain? Would M.S. make me mentally incapable? Ginsburg's reply to this question was only suggestive of an answer, and vague: "That's something we generally don't worry about." I interpreted this as there being a possibility, but it was extremely rare. And since he didn't worry about it, neither did I.

I had plenty of other questions to keep me occupied. Often I'd lay in bed at night just trying to organize the thoughts in my mind. Then, when Bob came, I'd ask him to write down my questions for me. But, when the doctor would arrive at the hospital, I'd seem to go mentally blank. I knew that I had many things to ask and that he had a schedule to keep, but I'd just forget my questions. I tried to get Bob to visit at the same time Dr. Ginsburg was there. My memory wasn't at its best and I didn't want to forget any information that was told to me. But, the doctor's time schedule varied and their meeting just didn't seem to work out.

So my written questions had to suffice. I wondered about many things now: Do people with M.S. drive? What should I do to check on the validity of my license? Did alcohol affect the disease? (Both Christmas and New Year's Eve were coming up.) What about smoking? Was there any special diet?

His answers were only good common sense. I should call the license bureau to make them aware of my disease and they would explain any special conditions which they would require.

It was very apparent that my present condition wasn't passable for a driver's license. My vision would have to improve about 90% before I could even find the car! I was told from the eye tests that I had blind spots and a loss of peripheral vision. I wasn't told if this condition would be permanent, but I assumed from remarks which I heard that it varied and probably wouldn't be.

Smoking and drinking weren't supposed to do any more or any less damage due to the disease. No special diet was prescribed. I was told that I could do anything that I felt like doing.

This wasn't so bad after all, a controllable disease with no restrictions. I was in no pain and had received an honorable discharge from my profession.

My attack actually provided an opportunity for me to see just how fortunate I am. Friends, family, love and concern were all there to help me. And I was going home, again.

But this time, rather than going from Olympia, Washington to Colorado, I'd be going from Rose Memorial Hospital to a real home, the home where I grew up. My husband and I had planned to stay with my mother during my recovery period. I'd be home for Christmas… and I planned to begin the New Year with a new appreciation for life.

Now that I knew what I had, I immediately began to call my family and friends, spreading the announcement of my new diagnosis. I was far from depressed, only relieved that they had found something to allow my early return home from Olympia in the middle of the booking. I now had a valid reason.

My explanations on the phone made me seem to have no more concern now, than if they'd discovered my problem to be only a common cold. I'd explain what was wrong with me and then I'd wait a silent minute while my other party recuperated. Generally their response was, "You sure seem to be handling it well. Just keep your spirits up!"

"Keep your spirits up!" That was all I heard for the next year. It seems that people generally agree that a positive attitude can produce miracles.

So far my spirits were up; my attitude was good. Even though I wasn't familiar with the disease, I was almost proud of its uniqueness. If I was destined to get an incurable disease, this one so far seemed all right. At least, it appeared to be something that I could handle emotionally.

I think Dr. Ginsburg was getting concerned about me for taking his diagnosis too easily. I presumed that he was worried about any adjustment problems which might come later.

But in my stoic style, I made an effort to suppress all self pity. My emotions broke down only once while I was in the hospital. I just needed to wash out my eyes a bit.

Ignorance makes it easy to be brave. I knew very little about M.S. My husband and brother had taken a crash course on their own with material supplied by Bob's cousin, a nurse. Bob had given me a general explanation of the disease and had supplied answers to some of my questions.

I was thankful for the information I had received and was determined to pursue information about the disease further as soon as my eyes allowed me to.

But, with time, I discovered that M.S. is characterized by exacerbations, called relapses, and remissions, periodic attacks that come and seem to go. This meant that I could have the problems that I was experiencing, recover to some degree of normality, and then possibly, start all over again.

It didn't take very long for me to realize that I didn't want to be responsible for this same situation reoccurring. My recovery wasn't progressing as rapidly as I had expected. So, we agreed that the duo would continue to entertain, change their name, their pictures, and their promotional material. I could still be involved with commercial production, writing, and even limited performing engagements. This solution answered an immediate need and still was possibly only temporary.

Before leaving the hospital, I had one more test, a bladder

examination. This was to be done in the surgical room of the hospital. I was given the full treatment this time, supposedly a going away present.

It began with a shot to relax, in needle form. Following this, I received a white gown and a green cap to cover my hair. (Only the cap covered my hair.) The next thing that I knew, they rolled a bed into my room and lifted me onto it.

This surgery procedure was beginning to worry me. I'd been told that this examination was minor, but I couldn't understand why it warranted relaxants and this cap build up. It was supposed to cost less if it was done in surgery rather than in a doctor's private office. So naturally, I preferred the hospital. But my rolling transport bed had arrived immediately after my shot. Things were happening a little too quickly for me. My shot hadn't taken effect. I was nevertheless rolled away, hoping that I would be aware of the medication by the time we arrived down at surgery.

At least I got a good look at the ceiling. That's all I could see passing by. But the hospital's biggest impression on me was the big swinging doors marked "SURGERY."

"Come on shot!" I didn't feel any different than when I'd left my room. Then, my bed was pulled up to a curtain and parked. I was left alone… to think, and presumably to relax.

Well, I didn't get tired, but I must have relaxed some. I'd even blink, and leave my eyes closed for a few seconds. But I remained generally alert. I certainly didn't want to miss anything! I thought mostly about the other people who, as I, were waiting for their turn; People quietly waiting, while sharing similar personal fears.

The examination turned out fine. As before, my doctor patiently explained the procedure to be done and some feelings which I might experience. (I had given up on my shot…) I felt alert and was never aware of the medication's effect.

But I became very aware of it afterward, as soon as I returned to my room. Now it was working! It may have been late, but it was effective. I was so dopey, all I could do was sleep.

I was supposed to go home that day, but I thought I'd take a little nap before calling Bob to come and get me. But understanding my earlier eagerness to leave, he and my brother, Roger, arrived quickly, just as I closed my eyes.

By now I was so dopey, I didn't even care about going home. I just wanted to sleep, but with their physical help and constant encouragement, I was packed and removed. I'm glad this decision wasn't dependent on my judgment. I might still be there...

Going home was a trip in itself. It was great to be out; I'd been in the hospital for about three weeks. Between tests, therapy, and sleeping, I'd lost track of the time. All I knew for sure was I had been there too long.

The air felt good; it was cold and stimulating. Bob had the car warmed up for me; the heater was on.

My poor eyesight contributed to the strangeness of my ride home. I felt as if we weren't moving, but the scenery was. It was strange and beautiful. At least the speed of the car wasn't frightening.

In all of the excitement about going home, I'd forgotten about my tiredness. But, I was totally relaxed when I finally got there, and I loved the drugged, tranquil feeling I was experiencing. I've always been considered a hyperactive person. At least, I have plenty of energy. But now, I could have been content to just sit in one place forever.

I seemed almost hypnotized at times. I'd catch myself staring at something - a wall, a person, or nothing in particular - but not really seeing anything. At least, nothing seemed to register mentally. It was like a fixation, lasting only a few seconds. I wasn't sure if it was noticeable to others, but neither they nor I said anything about my hypnotic state. Soon, I was encouraged to take a nap. I was still very tired and didn't object.

When I awoke, I was immediately anxious to get up, to get going, but I was quickly reminded that I was still dependent on help to get up, and my going had slowed down considerably.

But, it was great to be home! I'd slept quite a while but I still felt tired. This was just the beginning of my "sleep period." At first, I thought it was the medicine from the shot I'd gotten for my last hospital test, but when it continued for days, I wasn't sure what was causing it. But, I was too tired to be concerned. I seemed doped up, but I was taking nothing new. I had been getting two shots a day of ACTH, my miracle medicine, in the hospital and was supposed to continue with one shot per day for about a week longer. My family doctor had agreed to give me the shots daily at his office.

I was taking ACTH shots, (a)dreno (c)ortico (t)ropic (h)ormone. From my understanding, the hormone signals the body to produce more cortisone naturally and cope with stress. My only change had been, I was now taking one shot instead of two a day. I presumed this was less although I wasn't aware of the amount which was given.

Soon, I began to totally lose track of time. Days and nights became the same. I'd never slept so well in my life before! I never seemed to doze off. I was awake one second and asleep the next, as soon as I'd close my eyes. It was such a deep sleep. I seemed to be going deeper and deeper into a dark void.

I have always dreamed, but even that seemed to stop. At least, I had no awareness of dreaming. Nothing disturbed the heavy sleep. When I'd awaken, it seemed as though I was coming out of another world. I'd be up for a short time and then tired again. When awake, a feeling of total serenity was always present.

Unfortunately, this euphoric condition only lasted a few days. From then on my sensations became more and more peculiar. There seemed to be a constant pressure on my temples, as if someone was pushing in on each side of my head. I was thankful that it wasn't painful, only very annoying.

Then I thought that I could hear my heart beat. This wasn't bad until even it started acting strangely. At times two beats would be almost together, in rapid succession, like a heart palpitation. The noise of my heartbeat and the heavy pulsations in my temples discouraged me from lying on my side.

I had been asked in the hospital if I heard ringing noises. I hadn't … until now. What I heard wasn't actually ringing. A particular bass tone would tune in for a few seconds and then cut off. Then, there were some humming sounds- not tunes, but a single note. The noises weren't severe or loud, but were still very apparent.

The noises that were loud weren't coming from inside my head. Common, everyday, minor sounds were exaggerated into unbearable frustrating noises to me. I couldn't stand the sound of pots and pans in the kitchen, people talking, or even the sound of people walking down the hall. I didn't want to hear the television, or even any kind of music. It all seemed like confusion, which frustrated me. I desired my night-time void. I just wanted silence.

My equilibrium wasn't improving. In fact, if anything, it seemed worse. My head felt heavy, causing tiredness in my neck. I worried about losing control of the neck muscles that supported my head.

For some unknown reason, I also became very conscious of my tongue. Possibly it was numb, or maybe it was regaining feeling after having been numb, but I noticed a feeling at times, that I might swallow my tongue. I never choked or actually lost control of it, but I was aware of its presence and for some reason I developed this fear of losing its control.

When I asked my doctor about the possibilities of swallowing my tongue, I received the usual, indefinite answer, suggesting that I wouldn't.

My eyesight was going through its usual variations, throughout the day. Glasses couldn't even be considered due to the constant changes.

The numbness on the right side of my face reappeared periodically to remind me of its possible presence.

My bathtub storms continued.

But I still felt that I had been handling my new situation well; I wasn't feeling sorry for myself.

But then my disease turned in a new direction. The question which I had been concerned enough to ask about, the possibility of MS affecting the mind, began to answer itself. It seemed like my mind was running wild, out of control, as if it were a tape recording of memories being replayed on a fast speed. My thoughts were flighty, racing, and incomplete. I couldn't direct their progression, influence them, or even stop to rest.

Minor problems became exaggerated, like my noises. Solutions appeared impossible. My mind would jump irrationally from bits and pieces of unrelated subjects causing constant mental confusion. I remembered what I thought were forgotten words from songs I knew, and bits of past experiences in my life which had been apparently mentally recorded and filed. Nothing was complete enough to make any sense, but it made me realize that everything I do, is somehow being recorded mentally. It made me wonder why…

## Worth the Time

A man can spend his whole life chasing rainbows,
Just to finish, in the end, without a dime.
As they put him in a box made out of plywood,
Let them say, every dream, was worth the time.

A man can spend his whole life panning rivers
Growing weaker, day to day, 'til he's too old.
'til he falls beside his mine and drops his shovel,
Thinking still, one last try would find the gold.

If ever he should turn around and look at where he's been,
He'll find his scattered footprints on the ground.
Though they wander off in many ways
He can trace them back to golden days,
And think about the things he's never found.

If ever he should turn around and look at what he's left,
He'll find the scattered pages of the years,
Though they flutter off in many ways
He can trace them back to golden days,
With every fallen star, a dream appears.

A man can spend his whole life counting raindrops
Just to finish, in the end, without a dime.
As they put him in a box made out of plywood,
Let them say, every dream, was worth the time.

**Recording history: Fall River Records, Achilles solo album, 1975, Aspen Records,**
**F.A.B. Company, Our Songs For You, Illiad Publishing Co.**

# II

## Second Month

## December

Depression can be everyone's worst enemy. Trying to minimize its power, I have always tried to openly examine my problem before deciding on a course of action to choose for my defense. I generally end up comparing my problem to other peoples and then I realize that there are others worse off than myself, but now my usual defense had been lost. In my mental confusion, I was incapable of any kind of rational thinking. I only wanted to find the "stop" button, which would end the barrage of incomplete thoughts that constantly raced through my mind.

I was unable to organize my thoughts well enough to even begin to understand what my problem was. I was helpless against the depression, which enveloped my body as if it were a dark, heavy cloud. I couldn't rationally defend myself. Something was definitely affecting my brain...

I have never, before or since, felt so totally helpless in my life. I was helpless, both physically and mentally. I couldn't even go to the bathroom by myself! I couldn't stand up in a shower and I couldn't get in or out of a bathtub safely. I couldn't cook for myself or even see the numbers on the telephone, to dial someone, in case I needed help. I couldn't see well enough to put on any make up or well enough to miss it when it wasn't there. Simple functioning was difficult for me. Even brushing my hair, or my teeth became a new challenge.

Sure, I could do anything I felt like... but I didn't feel like doing anything, but sleeping. Sure, I could have children but who would care for them? With my depression, my physical and mental problems, my exaggeration of sounds, and my frustrations, I'd be afraid to trust myself around anyone's children, much less my own. I'd be afraid that I might harm them. In my mental derangement, I was capable of doing anything!

What kind of a future did this disease hold for me? The possibility of permanent physical disability and mental impairment seemed unbearable to me. What good was I now? Was this my fate, to only exist as a burden, a financial and physical problem for others?

I have always questioned and feared death. I realize that I am not unique; it is not unusual to fear death. The fear is questioning the unknown, the unfamiliar.

I guess I believe in a creator of life, but I can't accept that there is a personal type of god who is interested in my welfare. I feel too insignificant for any special consideration or concern. If I was created, I feel that I must have a purpose, a reason for living. But, I also believe that each person can only find the answers for himself.

I question the existence of a heaven. Although I don't disavow the possibility of life after death in some form, my present life is of great importance to me. It may be my only life…

But now I feared something new, other than death. I feared not dying. I feared living in my disabled condition. Me? How could I go on, confined to a bed and incapable of completing even simple tasks? Me? I couldn't even organize my own thoughts! Me? Would I be a living nothing, a vegetable, existing only to take from others while contributing nothing? I had changed and my fears had changed… I now desired to die.

I would lie in my bed, close my eyes and imagine a peaceful field in my mind. One lone, very old tree grew out of the lush green grass. I could visualize this place and longed to go there. The scene held a strange attraction over me, luring me to come…and I wanted to go. I wanted to lie down in the tall grass beneath the tree and sleep in my deep and peaceful rest. I desired the void that I had experienced, the nothingness to envelope me. For in my deep sleep, there were no worries, no concerns, no expectations, no fears…

Either my disease or the medicine was affecting my brain. And the escape which my field offered became very personal to me. Maybe I was going to die. I seemed to be so close, so near to the void.

I had no fear of dying now. In fact, I was anxious. And, I certainly wasn't concerned with other people. I felt as though I was beyond communicating with them.

I still loved my family and my friends, but I didn't have time to be concerned with them at this point. I seemed to be drifting in euphoria. I was there, and yet, not really there... aware of others, and yet, not interested or concerned with them.

I've since wondered if this state may be common before death. It seems to be interpreted as a sign that the patient is giving up, accepting his death. Could it be that this cold indifference to others, this quiet resignation while changing worlds, is planned and is a desirable, necessary, transition state?

My trance-like state continued after my ACTH shot series had ended.

These shot visits were educational. They made me realize that people generally form opinions from what they hear and see.

I'd enter my doctor's office being greeted with a comment like, "It seems you're walking better!" Walking was the least of my concerns. I was mentally a wreck! And, if I appeared to be walking better, it was only because I had someone to hold me up.

The most visible change did appear in my walking. But, the invisible mind changed without detection. It made me realize that I would never know what mental turmoil, pain, or depression was affecting others. Only the outward appearance is recognizable.

I worried about my friends. How would they be able to detect my mental condition? I found myself looking at people as though I were listening, and yet not mentally registering anything that was said. I was concerned about this lack of communication. For me, there seemed to be a link missing, a disconnection in my transmission of ideas. How would others interpret this if they talked and I merely acknowledged my agreement with a nod? Would I be accused of ignoring their conversation?

My equilibrium was still a mess and mentally I was confused and disoriented. I forgot things instantaneously. I'd say a sentence, and immediately ask what it was I had said.

One of the tests in the hospital had been repeating several

sentences after the doctor. At that time, this memory loss was not affecting me. Now, the hospital test that seemed so simple would be impossible.

I was now incapable of making even minor decisions. On one occasion at the doctor's office, I pulled my pants down to receive my ACTH shot, in my rear, while standing up. At the same time, the phone rang. My doctor was called to the phone, but gave me the injection first. He told me to wait there. My mental state on this day was so poor that my doctor's simple direction became a major decision for me.

I had been left leaning against the wall, my pants still down, and directed to stay there. My decision was whether or not I should pull my pants back up. Now this doesn't seem to be much of a decision. Pulling your pants up seems to be an automatic, natural reaction, but not to me. I was confused and didn't wish to ignore my doctor's request.

Somehow, I realized that this shouldn't be a major problem and I became frustrated with my own confusion. The harder I tried to decide, the more difficult my thinking became. My mind would go blank.

Finally, in desperation, I pulled my pants up. I had no idea if my choice had been correct, but at least it had been completed.

Christmas was getting close. In my usual style, I had waited until the last minute to buy gifts. This year the gifts would be "few and far between."

My brother, Roger, decided that I just wasn't in the old Christmas spirit this year and what I needed was to view the holiday lights, decorations, and shoppers, to bring my spirits up. Without my consent, I was supposed to accompany my husband, my sister, my brother and his fiancée on a Christmas shopping trip in a nearby shopping mall.

Before leaving the hospital, Dr. Ginsburg had warned me that I'd be very susceptible to colds or other common health problems and that it was very important for me to avoid these in my condition at that time. I wasn't interested in my Christmas spirit, but I was concerned about the possibility of contacting undesirable germs. I, with MS, was worried about others who might be contagious! You never know who you can trust these days...

I was very self-conscious about my disease. My only experience with sickness had been common, contagious illnesses, such as mumps, measles, chicken pox, or a common cold. My first normal reaction was to withdraw from people, fearing some possible transmission of the disease.

MS is considered not to be contagious. But, since no one is certain of its origin, its course, or its cure, it cannot definitely be stated that it is not contagious. At first, I felt no one should drink after me or even get very close to me. I reacted as if the disease was contagious. But, I soon decided that I was neither informed nor capable enough to make any new discoveries in MS.

My Christmas shopping trip took me into a large mall that had a fountain in the center. Chairs and couches were situated around the central fountain for those who needed to rest while spending their money. I didn't have any money to spend, but I did need to rest after limping in from the parking lot. Since I wasn't anxious to visit the stores, I was left to watch the fountain while my family finished their holiday shopping.

And, I would have enjoyed watching the fountain, or the people, if I could only have seen them. I began looking around, trying to analyze my visual problem, deciding what I could see. It seemed like an old time movie with motion breaks in the action which flickered on and off between picture frames. I decided that this was due to the blind spots which the doctor had told me about. In my effort to see, I ended up staring at people... until I realized that they were staring back at me...

There I was, quietly sitting at the fountain, trying to see, when an older woman, sitting next to me, attempted to begin a conversation. She evidently felt uncomfortable with us sitting so close together and not talking. I wonder what it is that disturbs people when they are close and yet quiet. It must be our animal instinct of protection, to be leery of others until some sign of acceptance is recognized.

Our strained conversation began with the general exchange of meaningless words about the condition of the weather. The uneasiness continued with long silent pauses between sentences. I could tell that my friend was working up to her big question of interest. I had limped over to my chair holding on to my husband on one side and trying to use my physical therapy cane on the other side. The conspicuous cane was now leaning against my chair.

My new friend politely asked if I had injured my leg. What she wanted to know was, what was wrong with me. My decisive moment had arrived. Would I ignore the woman's interest and belittle my diseased condition? Would deceiving her prevent any further discussion of my problem? Or should I accept the fact that I had an incurable disease and begin to acknowledge the truth?

I tried to do both, discourage and acknowledge. "I just got out of the hospital where I found out that I have Multiple Sclerosis." There, I'd said it. It seemed to me that she would now recognize the seriousness of my condition and leave me alone.

But, rather than discouraging her, this opened up a whole new topic of conversation. She proceeded to tell me that her sister has a friend who has MS, who also has a beautiful cane. I then received a full description of her carved piece of wood.

I wasn't impressed. My friend meant well, she was friendly, and just needed to find a listener. She was here visiting her daughter, her son-in-law and her grandchildren. Or maybe it was she lived here and her daughter's family was visiting. I seemed to have missed the details. I started looking around for Bob…

Anyway, I still worried about germs. There were so many people there. I just knew I'd end up catching something. Anytime someone sneezed or coughed, I was ready to hide under my chair!

My shoppers were slow. One of the group would occasionally stop by my area to see how I was doing. I was ready to go home which was no surprise to them since I didn't want to come in the first place. There were just too many people and too much noise and confusion for me. I think Roger was right… I just wasn't in the spirit of things this year…

After my one trip, I discontinued shopping mall visits…but there were presents to be bought and not much time until the big day. I had been excused from all obligations of Christmas this year. My husband and brother were now in charge.

They spent most of their time encouraging me to get out of the house. I was becoming more and more paranoid, afraid of other people. I imagine it is common to avoid associations with others due to embarrassment of physical abnormalities, but that wasn't it. I felt totally insecure. According to Funk and Wagnall's Desk Dictionary, "insecure" means: "1. Liable to break, fall, collapse, etc.; unsafe. 2. Troubled by anxiety and apprehensiveness; threatened." I guess my husband and brother were aware of my psychological fears. But still, I was encouraged to go with them when they shopped, even if I would only wait in the car. I felt much safer there and was not expected to participate in shopping mall conversations.

When I'd get tired of waiting, I'd often rest, close my eyes, or turn on the car radio for a change of pace. The radio never stayed on for very long though. It seemed to be only noise. I'd switch the stations often, trying to find something, but never really knowing what I was looking for. When a sad song would come on, I'd immediately begin to cry. I'd turn the music off and then, for no reason, begin to cry all over again. I didn't need a reason. I wasn't feeling sorry for myself. I wasn't feeling anything. I just felt like crying...

I'd try to give myself a pep talk, to straighten up before my husband returned to the car. Since my reason for crying was unexplainable, I wished to avoid the expected questioning.

But things weren't going so badly. At least I was getting out some. The car wait seemed to work out better... until I was again recognized as a possible listener.

This particular day, I had dozed off only to be awakened by a tap on the car window. I looked out to see someone carrying a large box. My first response was to roll down the window to see what was wrong. But my urgency quickly reminded me about my hand coordination problems.

As soon as I was able to open the window, the girl started into a five minute dissertation about the poor children in some foreign country. I just wasn't ready for this... I listened but couldn't mentally register anything. The only thing which did make a clear impression on me was her final sentence. She was evidently selling something in the box and concluded with the suggestion that if I didn't wish to buy any, they would appreciate a contribution. "They" apparently were the organization supporting the poor children somewhere.

By now, I almost seemed to be in a trance. I had understood so little and I didn't know how to reply. I was so confused. I wasn't even sure if there was a question. How could I begin to explain my refusal to help children? Did I need to explain? I couldn't seem to organize anything in my head, in order to even respond.

Finally, I blurted out that I'd just gotten out of the hospital and I didn't care for any. I then rolled the window back up. I felt so helpless. I couldn't even communicate properly. How would others interpret my short replies? My rudeness was not intentional. It was merely an effort to explain myself. I'm sure she never realized how mentally confusing she had been for me.

I tried to relax again closing my eyes; I was still tired. A few minutes later, I was aroused by another knock on the window. I opened my eyes to see a young man carrying a box which looked remarkably similar to my last visitor.

Wishing to avoid repeating my confusion, I simply looked out at him, through my closed window, smiled, shook my head expressing no, and closed my eyes again. This time, I'm sure, he was more confused than I was. I just wasn't in much of a contribution mood…

Finally, the shopping was completed, and the big day arrived… or the big day arrived which ended the need for further shopping. I remember this Christmas as a day of confusion, visiting people, and opening and closing presents.

It didn't seem like Christmas. I was still in my other world, in a daze. I felt bad about receiving presents when so little was given. But, I did have an excuse. Everyone seemed so concerned about me, asking how I was doing and then visiting to witness my condition for themselves. I only wanted to be left alone… Somewhere where it was quiet…

I didn't feel like celebrating. I didn't care whose birthday it was! After my interest in the hospital concerning alcohol's effect on MS, I wasn't even interested in a glass of wine. I didn't need anything this year.

Christmas is usually a special time for pictures. Every year millions of rolls of film are sold prior to the holiday and developed after the New Year begins. This year was no exception; surprise flashes kept blinding me throughout the holidays. Again, I just wasn't in the spirit of things. Pictures with forced smiles are never very encouraging.

I enjoyed my Christmas alone, more than a week later. By then, I was at least aware and able to quietly view the gifts around the tree. I didn't even recognize gifts that I had opened before. It seemed to be the first time I had seen them. For me, Christmas was a time of frustration. Now that presents had been distributed and visitations concluded, I could rest again.

I was extremely nervous; loud noises frightened me, quiet noises were also frightening. But this wasn't new to me since my diagnosis.

After Christmas, my problems included everything from my normal vision variations, my temple pulsations, the humming sounds, heart palpitations, exaggerations of noises, equilibrium difficulties, and mental confusion to some nausea and minor aches and pains. The pain was mostly in my head- a headache. But mine was a combination of headache and head pain located on the left side of my head and covering the left eye. It had been the right side of my body which had previously been affected. It seems as if I remember something I learned about the left side of the brain controlling the right side of the body, or vice versa, but I'm not sure.

I had been told not to take aspirin, but the pain in my head was increasing. My mother called Dr. Ginsburg for me. He was out of town so his associate returned the call. He suggested that I take some Tylenol, a substitute for aspirin that has proven to be less upsetting to the stomach. I took one pill.

I had hardly swallowed it when my nausea began. I was sick, really sick! I hadn't eaten all day due to my headache and was now vomiting continuously on an empty stomach. The strain was evident. My head pain increased more and more as I became weaker and weaker. I wasn't overly concerned with the nausea, but my head was "killing me"! Each strain to vomit increased the pain.

Then, without reason, the nausea cleared up, as suddenly as it had begun. My head pain was reduced to a slight ache soon afterwards. My stomach muscles were sore from the repeated vomiting, but it felt as though the sickness had been removed from my body. As if I had been under some kind of a spell, the sick feeling seemed to pass over me, hesitating for some time in the middle, but both beginning and ending abruptly. My Tylenol hardly had time to reach my stomach, before I became nauseated. I couldn't blame the medicine.

In addition to my headaches, my back wasn't feeling its best. It also ached. I felt like I had the flu, with all of my muscles aching. I thought I either had the flu or a truck had run over my back, bruising and straining all of my muscles. Apparently, my MS was working on the nerves in my back. The aches and pains seemed to vary as much as my eyes did, sometimes lasting only a few hours and other times, for the entire day. It seemed strange to experience what seemed to be a physical, body injury that was caused by a disease.

## <u>*Look at Me*</u>

*Look at me, look at me, look at me.*
*I am here...I am hungry,*
*I need, I need, I need,*
*Someone to see inside of me...*

*Look at me, look at me, look at me.*
*Can't you see...I am searching,*
*Teach me, teach me, teach me,*
*So I...can feel...*

> *Issues... I have, emotional scars...*
> *My addictions change...like racing cars...*

*Look at me, look at me, look at me.*
*Can you...fill up...the hole?*
*I must, I must, I must,*
*Try to gain control.*

*Look at me, look at me, look at me.*
*Slow me down so I can stop.*
*I'm tired, I'm tired, I'm tired,*
*Of reaching for the top... (chorus)*

# III

## Third Month
## January, 1974

My most difficult time was between Christmas and New Year's Eve. This was my major aches, pain, and nausea era. On New Year's Eve, I gave up all of my party invitations and celebrations in order to be in bed early. I was exhausted! Anyway, I wasn't particularly anxiously awaiting my first year since my new disease diagnosis.

On the big night, I slept until midnight and then was awakened to join my family in welcoming in the New Year. Entertainment was provided by my husband and my brother who had replaced their New Year's hats with ski caps and traditional noisemakers with pots and pans. They danced around the room, celebrating with others in Times Square on television, welcoming in the New Year at the appropriate minute. We shared a little wine, which I even tasted, and changed T.V. stations to view the the New Year's countdown several times. We finally ended up watching a rock concert, which I totally enjoyed. The people's excitement was contagious; their enthusiasm and smiles were a welcome sight for beginning a new year.

This year was an exception, compared to other New Year's Eves. For the last five in a row, I had been on a stage singing Auld Lang Syne. Then there were other years, even before that. This year, I had planned to take New Year's Eve off, to join the other people who are entertained... or who entertain themselves.

So I did. I took it off. But this wasn't exactly what I had planned...

After my headache, I seemed to be steadily improving. But, I was still helpless, unable to care for myself. I was at home with my mother and younger sister, Kellie, who was 12, but my mother worked each day from 10 in the morning until 7 each night. My brother and his fiancée, Ann, were on their Christmas vacation from Colorado State University. Ann gave up going home to Boston for the holidays to join Roger in taking care of me. They both moved down to my mother's house to help out.

Meanwhile, Bob organized a moving party and we were officially moved out of our apartment in Boulder, and moved back home to Mom's.

Financially, we were in a mess... Following my diagnosis, Bob immediately dropped out of graduate school to find a job. Realizing the seriousness of my condition, he contacted a private security business which he had considered at an earlier time. He was accepted, and started to work.

Now, he had me to worry about plus adjusting to a new job and learning their procedures. He wasn't home much at first. The training period demanded much of his time, so, I was generally left in the care of my sister, Kellie, and Roger and Ann. I was thankful that someone could be there...

My only complaint was their over-concern about me. Things were carried to an extreme. If I was trying to sleep, everyone would whisper so they wouldn't bother me, but the whispering bothered me even more than if they were talking! Everyone seemed to be trying so hard, trying to adjust to my situation, to understand and be helpful. They were trying too hard.

Strong, individual personalities in the house seemed to conflict. We ended up having "too many chiefs and not enough Indians". Each person had different ideas, felt capable of handling my situation, and for some reason, thought that the others needed their strength and direction in this time of crisis. My mother, brother, Ann and Bob each seemed upset about me and each felt compelled to organize the confusion which resulted from their four, independent directions.

Meanwhile, I, the cause of all this confusion, lay in bed, helpless. I couldn't organize a plan for myself and certainly couldn't direct the others. Their intentions were good; the result was misunderstandings.

You can't mask emotions or discontent with words. A superficial pleasantness was displayed for the benefit of me, but there seemed to be a pervading ill feeling. Possibly, I imagined this, but, helplessly feeling the frustration, I also felt responsible. I worried that this strained situation might cause problems between my brother and Ann. I wondered about the ill feelings which might develop between Ann and my mother.

Kellie was also being affected by my disease. She would get upset and cry easily. It was evident that she was feeling a lack of attention. And, I blamed myself...I realized that I was the cause of all these problems. There didn't seem to be an answer. I only tried to avoid the frustration.

Bob's job was a necessity. He needed something secure which we could depend on, but now he was at work more than he was home. I was jealous. I was without him at the time when I needed him the most. Bob was stuck in the middle, without a choice; we both recognized the necessity of some kind of financial support.

I was frustrated... with myself, with my family, and with Bob's job. I worried about him... I wondered if his job was merely providing him with an escape from reality, my disease and the problems at home. I wondered if he would ever be able to understand my feelings and emotions. Could he understand what I had been through when he was gone? He seemed to be home so little...

How could we grow closer together when we were separated because of financial necessity? I wondered... and worried... and just wanted him to be with me. When he was home, I'd try to let him know how I felt, how much I needed him, but I would generally end up crying rather than explaining anything, and I knew this was wrong.

I tried to understand the pressure he was under and I didn't wish to add to his frustrations. I only wanted someone who could share my experience with me, someone who could understand how I felt. Everyone was trying... but I guess I desired the impossible.

My brother and Ann provided my major emotional outlet. Ann took over nurse duty, helping me whenever necessary. She was my cook, my exercise encourager, and my discussion partner. In her most important role, she was also my listener... It seemed very important to me at that time, to try to express my feelings and my experiences.

Since Roger and Ann were stuck with me more often than anyone else, they became my listeners.

Roger also volunteered for other positions. He appointed himself to organize morale booster sightseeing drives. Naturally, he provided his own original humor on each trip.

Then, there were my exercises… Both Roger and Bob were strong supporters of this program. I had been told that I needed to use my muscles, to redevelop them. I didn't understand why the muscles were important when I could hardly move my arm and my leg. But these guys weren't as understanding as my hospital P.T.s and they were determined that I <u>would</u> exercise.

So, Roger started out demonstrating the proper ways for me to fall. (It's always encouraging to begin with others expecting failure) but my right arm and leg were so weak that it was impossible for me to have any confidence in myself. I was afraid of falling, and afraid that I couldn't catch myself to break the fall. Roger compared my exercising to skiing, I'd have to learn how to fall, first.

My expectations and fears were soon confirmed. My leg was not only weak, but it had actually shrunk; the muscles were nothing but flabby tissue.

I also realized the need for reconditioning. I'd received two mimeographed exercise sheets from P.T., my suggested daily program, but I had been unable to begin due to tiredness and my sickness. By the time I thought I might be able to begin, I still couldn't see well enough to read the instructions. Ann and Kellie volunteered to read and interpret the exercises for me. Since my loss of memory had occurred, I was having trouble remembering how to do each exercise from day to day. So, my exercises varied, depending on the individual who read the instructions and their understanding of the directions. At least I was offered a diversified program.

As my improvement slowly continued, my natural impatient reaction was to attempt more than I was actually capable of doing; I decided to devise my own exercises which were more demanding. One of my personal exercises began with me laying down on my back with my legs extended straight up. Then, I would slowly lower them together, down to the floor. My leg and arm still felt heavy, but

I had designed this exercise to offer more of a challenge than the therapist's program.

Unfortunately, this one seemed a little too challenging for me. With stomach muscles tight, I strained to control my legs, lowering them together slowly. Everything was proceeding well when suddenly my right leg became anxious to return to the floor. It dropped straight down. Ugh...

It felt like I had pulled a muscle in my hip. My leg hurt, and my feelings were hurt; I was discouraged... I lay there, on the floor, trying to recuperate from my failure. Fortunately, nothing seemed to be permanently damaged, nothing but my pride...

That wasn't my first, and it wouldn't be my last failure. But I was determined to do my best, to regain my muscle strength. To be weak, underdeveloped, or not using the body to its fullest potential, seemed almost sinful to me, just an acceptance of life, ignoring its capabilities.

I now understood why the therapists at the hospital talked so much. Simple maneuvers now exhausted me. When in the hospital, my energy level was much higher; I was able to do more than they had asked of me. Now I needed to stop and rest every few seconds. Their conversation time had been designed as an unidentifiable rest period. Their program was just a little early for me.

But I continued to try to do as much as possible, and more, that was impossible. Improvement was slow. At least, it seemed slow to me. I tried to understand the need for exercising, and yet, it only frustrated me. It made me realistically aware of what I could not do. Lacking my visible progress, exercising became discouraging.

I knew it was important for me to use my muscles, to retain their flexibility, but I also knew that the muscle's use depended on the reparation or replacement of the nerve damage. If the nerve was dead, messages couldn't be transmitted properly to the muscle. The muscle would be useless; there would be no use for exercising. Since nerve damage can only be determined with time, my exercise program would continue until permanent nerve damage could be identified.

My understanding was that if I gave up exercising, I might somehow lose the muscle control. I also was under the impression that damaged nerves may be replaced by others which volunteer their help in chosen areas of the body.

When you break a leg, the bone needs time to heal, the cast is removed, the leg is shrunken, and the muscles are weak. Exercise is necessary for rebuilding its strength. There is visible progress.

With MS, my leg muscles were similar to someone who had just had a cast removed, but I had additional problems concerning its control. Exercising was important, yet there was no visible progress.

Initially, I had approached my disease with a determination to adjust to my new situation and to do everything possible to overcome my physical and emotional problems. Since that time, I now realized my inability to combat either of them successfully. I could control neither my mental state nor my body.

I felt so helpless... so insignificant... My body and my mind, were not mine to control. Their direction and my future was beyond me... and seemed to be beyond the doctors'. Someone, or something, was directing my course. I merely existed... for this unknown direction.

Time was very confusing to me. I slept a lot, and struggled with the reality of my disease when awake. I was mentally confused, and physically incapable. Because of my confusion and the disease vacillation, it was difficult for me to express my improvement by time or specific dates. I only knew that my recognizable symptoms began about the first of November and it was now getting close to February.

Improvement was slow. The continuation of my progress seemed as sporadic as my eyes. Exercise accomplishments of one day were often impossible achievements for the next. Each day was different. My condition depended on the inflammation of the nerves. When inflamed, the message was not properly transmitted.

Exercising was only one of my discouragements. My disease made me appreciate things which I had generally taken for granted. My eye problems made me realize how dependent I was on my vision. I couldn't see big or little things properly, but the small ones seemed to be more distressing. As my sight improved, I could tell that my eyebrows looked like one hairy mass, but I couldn't see well enough to pluck them as I had always done. I also had trouble cutting my fingernails. Try that sometime with your eyes closed.

I was still anxious to see well enough to read, to discover the real facts about MS. I wondered if information was being withheld from me, for my own benefit. Most of my questions were answered by Dr. Ginsburg with one statement, "We'll just have to wait." I wasn't sure what we were waiting for, but I didn't have much of a choice to do anything other than wait. I wasn't able to do much. So, I waited…

I continued to push myself and, as soon as I was able, I was up and hopping. By the end of the third month, I slowly began exercising daily and feeling better overall. My mental confusion was less and my depression seemed to be normal, but my emotions still continued to vary. I could wake up in the morning and tell if I was depressed or felt normal, before I even got out of bed. There was a definite division, a personal emotional state of mind. I finally learned to remain in bed to avoid others when I was aware of my depressive moodiness.

Anxious to be self- dependent again, I ventured into the kitchen one afternoon to warm something for my lunch. I was proud of my improvement and any minor accomplishments for my condition. I think that it was soup which I was preparing for my afternoon meal. I decided that I'd try to keep the kitchen clean on my first cooking attempt, so I began to wipe off the stove. I not only wiped off the porcelain top, but I decided to clean up the burners. It never occurred to me that the burners were hot! At least, it didn't occur until my dishcloth started smoking.

This scared me! Fortunately, the cloth never flared up into flames, but it frightened me to think that I wasn't aware of little things which I had previously taken for granted. This had been senseless! I thought that I could wipe off a hot burner! And yet, I was unable to comprehend any danger in my confused state of mind. My danger connection had been disconnected. This inability to make decisions or to comprehend danger showed me how vulnerable I was to injury.

My first doctor visit came and went in about 45 minutes. This was my first office appointment with Dr. Ginsburg since his hospital visitations. My understanding of my disease was still as vague as the last time I had seen him. My appointment was scheduled for approximately a month and a half after my ACTH shot series had ended. I couldn't see, I still limped, and I experienced my depression and nausea alone, without my physician's observation. His only awareness of my difficult period had been one telephone call questioning headache medication during my nausea period. Even then, he'd been out of town, and his associate had responded to my call. I had only talked to Dr. Ginsburg once since then.

I felt as though I was pretty much on my own, but my doctor provided my only hope; my destiny was in his hands. I didn't know how I could begin to relate my experiences to him, which had occurred since he had seen me last.

Being a professional entertainer makes you become very leery of people at times. It's easy to lose faith in promises and become very mistrusting. It always seems that nothing gets done, unless you do it yourself. But, now I was in a situation which depended solely on the decisions of another individual… decisions which I was incapable of making. And these decisions were not minor to me. My life depended on them!

Decisions are dependent on a knowledge of the facts affecting the situation. I felt responsible for providing those facts. I wanted Dr. Ginsburg to realize that he had only observed me when I was feeling my best. I wanted him to understand what I had been through in the interim, since I had seen him last.

Understandably, all patients must experience similar fears and believe that their case deserves special attention, and I assume most doctors have to understand these common fears which their patients experience. My fear made me lose all self-confidence and left me clinging with total dependency on another, my doctor. I wanted him to understand. My case may not have been different, but it was special. It was very special to me…

His questions were short and direct. His answers were general and open to personal interpretation. I supplied most of the questions and he provided most of the answers, which I interpreted to my liking. (Doctors must have a special required course in suggestive answers while not jeopardizing themselves.)

I had plenty of questions: Can you tell anything from the severity of the attack? Can you predict my future condition? Does the initial attack indicate future progression? Were my experiences common? Was my attack minor, normal or extreme when compared to others diagnosed with MS?

While I was in the hospital, my cholesterol count had been high. Was this common with MS? Was there any particular diet which I should follow? Was my nausea due to the disease or was it caused by the food I had eaten? What was his opinion of the Denver Chapter of the Multiple Sclerosis Society of Colorado? Did he agree with the Low Fat Diet, which they highly recommended? What about special vitamins? Can excessive exercise and over tiring be harmful? Would he suggest other pain medication other than Tylenol for my headaches? How could I determine if I had an infection in my bladder or kidneys, or if the nerves were only being affected from the MS? Were my headaches and nausea an indication of a turning point in my attack? Do patients build to a particular peak and then begin to improve?

My last questions pertained to the ACTH shots. Dr. Ginsburg had explained to me that there were a number of different drugs, which were used to combat the disease. If one medication proved helpful in an attack, it didn't necessarily mean that it would work equally as well the next time. He explained that he could try several, and asked me not to become discouraged if there seemed to be few positive results after his first attempt.

I had taken the ACTH shot series for two weeks, which was considered a trial period. If this was the length of a common trial period, how many varieties of control did he have to offer? It seemed to me that the patient could spend the most critical time experimenting, trying to find the drug that would work.

I had been told that MS was not curable, but it was controllable. Was this the control? If the disease is characterized by reoccurring attacks, exacerbations or relapses, and periods of recovery, remissions, how could he determine if a certain medication was helpful or if the course of the unpredictable disease was merely entering its remission stage? Using this same understanding, the same drug might appear to be of no help if the exacerbation hadn't reached its turning point. My question was, how could you differentiate between the effect of the shots and the effect of the disease? Could you determine if it's the medication or the course of the disease which attributes to any improvement? If attacks or spells occur often, was the patient supposed to be under continuous observation and constant medication?

My drug questions were all directed toward acquiring one answer. Was MS really controllable? I didn't understand how it possibly could be. How could anyone control a disease if they didn't know its origin, its cause, its progression, and its unpredictable variations. I had built my own case in an effort to find the truth, a case which could destroy my only hope for this incurable disease.

I respect Dr. Ginsburg for his honesty. Although his answers were often not direct, he was truthful with me. When confronted with my not curable but controllable questions, he responded with the fact that there are medications that doctors use for treatment of the disease.

A dictionary definition of "control" is "to exercise authority or dominating influence over: direct; regulate." Therefore, a controllable disease would be one that doctors could influence or regulate. Their only verification of this control is statistical information on the effects that different drugs have had on MS patients.

So the disease was "not curable, but controllable." I explained my misunderstanding of the word controllable. It seemed to me that Dr. Ginsburg had given several misleading answers. Or were they only misleading to me? Could it be that I interpreted the answers as I wanted them to be? Maybe I wasn't even coherent enough to understand his explanations at the time…

I forgot so many things. Dr. Ginsburg would calmly repeat himself following the reminder, "As I told you before", or "We have discussed this earlier." He was never harsh, always patient, but wanting to emphasize the importance of my listening to his explanations.

I felt very small. I knew that he was an intelligent, highly recommended neurologist. I knew that his time was valuable, and I knew that this repetition thing was getting out of hand. I didn't want to feel responsible for using other people's time, neither other patients' or the doctor's. He was so patient…a good lesson for me.

Dr. Ginsburg spoke of steroids when explaining his control. I got the impression that these were drugs that were used commonly as control treatments for MS. The medications were strong, commonly had undesirable side effects, and were used sparingly to avoid danger to the body. Periods of two weeks duration of treatment seemed about average. I'm not certain about the minimum amount of time necessary to determine possible improvement.

My major question had been answered. MS is controllable by treatment, but there is no way for the doctors to determine if it is the medication, or the course of the disease, which is responsible for the improvement.

They didn't know... they weren't sure... Nothing seemed to be definite; there were no real assurances... The doctors were aware of the effects of the medication; they were knowledgeable about its influence on the body, but research and statistical results were their only measurements. So, I had a controllable disease, while no one could definitely verify that my prescribed treatment was responsible for my improvement.

Why hadn't I been told this from the first? Why was this false hope encouraged? It was my body, my disease, my decisions on how to handle my personal situation! I wanted truth, honesty and definite answers!

Dr. Ginsburg reassured me that he was supplying those exact things. He explained the fact, that I, or anyone who has an incurable disease, is initially a big adjustment in itself. The statement that MS is controllable is a fact. To follow the announcement of the diagnosis with pessimism would only add to a patient's emotional problems.

As long as he was honest with me, I was satisfied. It would now be up to me to ask the right questions that would supply informative answers.

His other answers were less definite: Yes, the exacerbation can build to a type of peak condition. The improvement stage is termed a remission. The nausea may have indicated a turning point; everyone is different. Kidney and bladder infections can be determined by a urologist or doctors other than himself. There were no significant tests which could be done at home. Tylenol was sufficient medication for minor pain, although other pain pills could be prescribed if necessary. He suggested that I shouldn't enter the Olympics but I could run around the block if I felt like it. Dr. Ginsburg restated his philosophy that I could do anything that I felt like doing. But this time, he suggested that I shouldn't "overdo" things or go to any extremes in my self-testing program. He advised me to try activities in moderation and then build up. Nothing had been proven to discourage exercise.

Dr. Ginsburg isn't a strong vitamin proponent. He left that up to me. If I felt as if I was deficient in a certain vitamin, I should take it; a multiple vitamin was suggested. In the same manner, he didn't particularly encourage the MS Society's Low Fat Diet. He didn't discourage it either. Again, that was my decision. He did recognize the Society's contributions to MS; he felt that the opinions of different MS state societies seemed to vary as widely as the disease itself.

He didn't feel that my nausea resulted directly from the MS. He suggested no particular diet for me, but warned that people with MS tend to be overweight due to inactivity. I could easily understand how physical limitations could restrict activity. I was told that high cholesterol had nothing to do with MS. He suggested that my attack had the normal characteristics common to MS patients. This was another one of his safe answers. And, finally, no, nothing could be determined by the first attack; it did not indicate future severity or progression of exacerbations.

Dr. Ginsburg had told me in the hospital that I would just have to wait, and apparently that was only the beginning of my waiting. He sounded as helpless as I, in predicting what I could expect to occur. I'm sure that he could have told me what might occur, but why should he suggest possible problems? I agreed with this idea, whether it was intended or not. It saves the patient from unnecessary worry. There are plenty of other things to worry about... and besides, everyone is different; nothing can be definitely determined for individual cases.

Even following my initial dissatisfaction with Dr. Ginsburg's answers, I still respect the man. I began to realize that beyond his medical knowledge, he was supposed to diagnose the disease and also act as a psychological advisor and personal psychiatrist. His attitude, his response, his answers could be helpful or emotionally harmful to his patients. This seemed to be more responsibility than I could conceive of. Respect and admiration is all that I can offer to Dr. Stanley Ginsburg and others like him who offer their knowledge, their ability, their time, and their emotions to help people like me.

Everyone needs self- discipline. I know that I need a direction, a definite course of action to follow, a goal which I desire to achieve. People complain about work, and yet, generally I think they would be lost without it. There seems to be a need in each of us for personal achievement. Each definition of achievement varies according to the individual, but the need for accomplishment seems to be desired by all.

At least, it is desired by me. Competition has been my encouragement in sports, in talent, and in the entertainment business. Winning was the desired achievement. Unfortunately, it became synonymous with accomplishment.

As soon as my physical and mental condition began to improve, I automatically began to set up a definite pattern of desired goals, which I wished to complete. This occurred even before my father encouraged a similar goal-oriented program for me to follow. (I wonder where I got my idea?)

Inherited or learned, free will is beyond me... Directed and programmed from a very early impressionable age, I am definitely a product of my parents.

My desires at this time may have seemed insignificant to others, but I felt compelled to achieve them. It must have been an attempt to regain normality, get going again, not an effort to erase my disease. I didn't want to concentrate on my illness. I needed to be busy, and, significant or not, there seemed to be plenty to do.

Since my parents were divorced, our furniture ended up at my dad's, while the majority of the boxes were at my mother's house. They were stacked in the basement with no one knowing what, or where, or in which box articles were located. Since my husband had been responsible for packing and moving, I knew that I would be in charge of organizing and locating the articles.

I wasn't immediately frustrated with my inability to begin this task, but I was concerned about cleaning. Bob and I had moved into my old bedroom in the basement, and I felt in charge of keeping it at least livable.

My equilibrium seemed to be improving, but it still was not normal. So, that offered me quite a challenge, such as climbing up on a chair to vacuum the windowsill of our basement bedroom. Climbing up wasn't difficult, but standing up was... Realizing a tendency to perceive motion in the room, I was particularly careful. Careful, but determined to clean!

Anything that indicated the use of any energy resulted in great fatigue for me. Regardless of how minor the activity was, I was exhausted. I was taking no medication at the time, so I had nothing to blame my tiredness on except the disease. I'd awaken feeling well and full of good intentions, anxious to assume daily household chores. I'd begin vacuuming. I'd start to vacuum our tiny bathroom and would be too tired to continue cleaning the sink or the toilet. At this pace, this amounted to endless cleaning and discouragement!

I'd begin rearranging the boxes in the same manner, beginning enthusiastically, completing what was possible for me each day, and finally finishing, proud of my accomplishment.

Then there were ordinary housewife duties. Although I'd been married for three years, I didn't actually consider myself a "housewife", at least not in the traditional sense. My husband had been left pretty much on his own.

I am not a good cook and I don't sew. I don't cook breakfast, for anyone, and I'm not interested in learning how. Fortunately, I have been able to afford to eat out.

I've always bought all of my clothes. I don't have the patience to sew. While entertaining, I was usually still in bed, while my husband ate breakfast. I felt that he was capable of getting his own breakfast and achieving his own accomplishments without my personal, continuous praise. I'm a poor actress for playing the supporting roles to the man I married.

I probably wouldn't be considered the ideal wife... Entertaining can be a demanding profession. I was up late at night, often followed by business meetings at breakfast. There were rehearsals, recordings and meetings with club owners, agents and prospective commercial clients, travel, personal promotion, and a million other time consuming efforts to direct and promote the group's career.

For a woman, it leaves little time for having babies, and too often, little time for your husband. I was business, not housewife oriented, so ordinary housewife duties were a new experience for me. I was generally accustomed to spending very little time at home. My past wifely duties had consisted of some housecleaning, preparing an occasional meal, throwing some clothes into the washer or dryer, and dropping the others off at the dry cleaner's. I didn't wash or iron any of Bob's shirts or any of my own dresses.

But now I had new problems to confront; health and financial problems which I was suddenly incapable of directing. At least I could help to reduce the dry cleaning bill. I decided to wash and iron Bob's shirts. I did have one thing now which I had never had before... time.

The washing went well, the ironing went slowly. I did discover that washing and ironing gives a woman plenty of time for thinking. Neither takes concentration; each allows time for daydreaming. I wasn't very enthusiastic about my new duties. There was no intrigue. But it was necessary, and I was accomplishing something. Bob was great: he never complained.

Cleaning was an accomplishment, but I did need some time out of the house, so I decided to take walks... My limp was still very obvious to others; the heaviness of my leg was obvious to me alone, but it was great to be outside! Sickness and confinement to a bedroom made me appreciate the beauty and freedom that was outside. Everything looked, felt and smelled beautiful and different. Colors appeared more vivid, smells were more distinctive. I thought that I could even hear better! At least I was more aware of sounds. All of my senses seemed to be more acute.

I began my walking by going down the block a short way and back again. I couldn't go far because of my tiredness. Then, after some time, I slowly progressed to walking around the block. That was a journey!

I couldn't see very clearly. I had lost a great deal of my peripheral vision. As I walked, I couldn't see my legs or my feet. Everything else was blurry. On top of that, I had no distance perspective.

Nothing was distinct or discernable. My legs seemed to move voluntarily forward, automatically carrying me. I felt like I was floating, or being carried in some invisible machine. The heaviness in my arm and leg became emphasized with the walking. The longer I walked, the worse my vision became.

I sometimes felt as though I was split down the center of my body. The right side felt as though it was either dying, or already dead. The left half felt alert and alive. I knew that the right side existed, but it was not useful. My body seemed to be battling itself with a clear division between the left and the right sides. The right side was diseased, tired and heavy, pulling me back constantly. The left side pushed forward, reaching out for normality, dragging the sick half of my body.

My walks, like the exercises, were discouraging at first, but I knew that the exercise was important for my weak leg muscles. I looked down a lot while walking. There was nothing to look up for; I couldn't see well enough. I could only distinguish a mass of colors, blurriness and movement. No one understood why I wasn't interested in sitting inside, by a window, where I could look out. But when you can't see properly, it definitely limits your looking!

I wasn't interested in going for rides either. I liked to be outside, but not particularly in a car. And, because MS creates a false feeling of movement or motion, I had no desire to go faster; I was going faster than anyone else already on my own personal trip!

When I'd walk around the block, my right leg would always begin to ache behind the knee. Possibly it was due to some damaged nerves in that area, or the added strain on nerves which had replaced others in the injured area.

A daily walk became one of my goals to accomplish. Finally, I worked up to a new achievement; I hiked three blocks to the store where my mother worked. I got there… but I wasn't feeling my best. In fact, I felt weak, lightheaded, and faint. My leg ached, my vision was blurred and confused, and I was exhausted, but I got there…

Again, I was discouraged and disappointed in my body's response to walking three blocks. When I had started, I felt great! I was proud of my progress, and felt optimistic about my personal disease case. After my walk, my thinking had changed. What could I do, when only three blocks was too far for me to walk?

So, instead of walking, I decided I should try jogging. I didn't go far, and I didn't go fast, but I attempted to include jogging in my daily exercise. I only knew that it might strengthen my leg. When you can't join them, beat them! At least, that was my new philosophy.

I'd begin with my usual walks, and then jog a little along the way. I wasn't sure if it was strengthening my leg, but the other effects were apparent. The activity caused the same old mental confusion, faintness, visual blurriness, and aching sensations in my arm or leg or both. These, like my other MS characteristics, varied daily, but I was anxious to achieve some type of near normality.

As soon as I was more confident about my equilibrium in walking and jogging, I decided bicycle riding would be good for me. At least it would be challenging! I was a little more leery of this. Both my equilibrium and my vision were still poor, but I knew it would be good for my leg muscle development. Anyway, all I could do was fall!

I carefully got on the bike in my mother's driveway... and, not so carefully, fell off before I even reached the street. Things were a bit shaky. The cement wasn't as soft as I had remembered it to be years ago, and, at twenty-five, I was too old to be crashing into pavements! But it had only been my first try. If I could only avoid breaking any bones or seriously injuring myself, maybe I could still do it. I felt that I just needed another chance.

I remounted my Schwinn to try again. This time I fortunately stayed on... not confidently, but miraculously. I had persuaded my sister to ride her bike with me. Since I still couldn't see, she was my leader, responsible for identifying hazards like walls, curbs or cars.

We ventured all the way around the block... and my right leg knew it! It was so tired. It felt as if it had died. My vision also affected my judgment of speed. As in the car, I was still unable to tell if I was moving. Even I could recognize the danger involved in this, so I tried to hold the speed of my bicycle down. I think I was going somewhere between slow and slower. No wonder I had trouble staying up.

I soon realized that my poor vision affected everything I did. Everything was blurry and I was unable to judge distance. For a little arm exercise, I attempted a few shots with the old basketball one day. I was lucky to locate the rim, but judging the distance to the basket was impossible. I decided to hold off for a while before trying out for any professional teams...

Each time that I was defeated, each time that I couldn't accomplish what I had intended, I expected my defeat to be permanent. I never thought if I can't walk three blocks today, maybe I'll be able to do it tomorrow… All I knew for sure was that I couldn't do it today and I might never be able to progress any further. I might be losing my optimistic approach.

Patience… that's what Dr. Ginsburg prescribed, but it's always easier to be patient about someone else's condition.

# <u>I Can't Love You Enough</u>

© *1972 Bonnie Lynne Ellison / All Rights Reserved*

*Let's take the day off, stay in bed...*
*You look so good in the morning...*
*Peacefulness is all around us,*
*But I can't love you enough.*

    *I can't love you enough, to make you,*
    *Understand me, like I do.*
    *And I can't love you enough, to make me,*
    *Understand, why I love you...um, umm*

*Do you think, that we, could get much closer?*
*You lay beside me in the morning.*
*Your body feels so warm and tempting,*
*But I can't love you enough.*
    *How can I tell you,*
    *How much I need you,*
    *Will you ever know? (music)*
*Maybe I'll never find the answer.*
*Maybe we'll never understand.*
*What makes a man, desire one woman,*
*Why does a woman need her man?*

*(chorus) I don't know the reason, but I do...love you...yes, I do love you*

# IV

**Fourth Month**

**February**

At this stage, I had something which everyone desires... time. I couldn't do much, but no one expected much. Organizing boxes, washing and ironing, folding clothes, and straightening the bed each day allows a lot of thinking time. My thinking time wasn't particularly creative. It was more worry-oriented. Housewife duties may be time consuming, but they're not what I call "attention getting". Daily necessities may be completed while the mind wanders off on a separate journey. With the awareness of an incurable disease added to my mental confusion, my household daydreaming was not particularly optimistic.

I was primarily concerned with my husband's adjustment to my condition, and how our relationship would be affected. Bob's new job was demanding of his time. He was going through some initial training procedures to obtain a specific management position. The difference in mental pressure, from graduate school to trying to achieve a needed financial goal to support the two of us, was evident.

Meanwhile, I was far from well. I cried easily... I didn't need a specific reason for depression or crying. I told Bob that I had weak eyes... Realizing that it was not a good idea to have my husband come home to find me crying every other night, I worried about his reaction. I tried to have more control, but control seemed helpless. Bob comforted me the best he could. I knew he didn't understand why I was crying... but neither did I...

The questions that worried me the most were impossible to answer. I wondered about my future... Would this condition which I was experiencing now become my new normality? Should I expect to continue to be emotionally depressed? Was this high fatigue normal with MS? Would I continue to improve, at least mentally? Or, should I accept the disease, expecting another attack?

I, along with others, knew very little about MS. But, I thought I knew a little more about men. Singing in nightclubs for six years can be very educational. Since I had returned home from the hospital, I had gone through a time when I couldn't control my coordination properly in my right arm, hand or leg. My nerves were bad. I had trouble even turning over in bed. I was experiencing great fatigue and depression, I was mentally confused, and emotionally, I was of little help to anyone.

Beyond this, I had no interest in sex with my husband. In fact, I had no interest in sex with anyone! Physical disability was one thing, but this was entirely new for me! I was generally overly aggressive sexually. Entertainers tend to have large egos which desire compliments and acceptance to be satisfied.

Everyone needs to prove himself as a man or woman sexually. Physical disability and mental disability from a disease do not suggest sexual dysfunction. This seemed to be the last straw! Was this common with MS? Now, I was too tired or too upset to make any attempt to make love.

I've always been extremely jealous, but now I was concerned about his desires. I never encouraged "extra marital activities" but my jealousy had changed to a personal concern for him.

Bob had once told me that my disease would only make us grow closer together. Now, I was beginning to question that. How could he ever understand how I felt… how could anyone?

I'll always remember the first time that I went to a local discotheque after my disease diagnosis. I won't mention the club's name, but I think it originated from their clientele and the social games which people play. I've always enjoyed dancing. I guess I was only reaching for the old reality which I remembered.

The scene was typical of a club for young people, offering loud music, alcohol, and an opportunity to meet other attractive young people, but this time, nothing seemed the same. It seemed like another world to me, a world removed from the disease, and the life and death realities which I had experienced. Everyone laughed and smiled outwardly. It reminded me of my lesson at the doctor's office: I now realized that their outward expressions were no indication of their inward personal struggles. There seemed to be a lot of loneliness hidden behind their smiles.

I didn't dance. I only watched the other people. I couldn't find my old reality. In fact, the club seemed to be an escape from all reality... possibly, a very necessary escape at times...

# Easy Lovin' Day

Nice day, for a walk in the park,
Watchin' things grow.
Nice day for your head movin' fast,
While you're movin' slow.

Easy rush of warmness,
Flowin' inside of me,
Takin' in some country,
Right here in the middle of the city.

> Nice day for a walk in the park,
> Easy lovin' day...

Nice day, for feelin' the grass,
Layin' under the trees,
Nice day for smellin' the green,
Blowin' in the breeze.

Children sharin' secrets,
With new friends they've found,
Runnin' through the sprinklers, with their puppy dogs,
Playin' with imaginary clowns.

> Nice day for a walk in the park,
> Easy lovin' day...
> > La da da da da dad a...
> > La... Easy, lovin' day...

Nice day, to drift with the clouds,
Into the blue,
Nice day, to sail high on a kite,
Makin' dreams come true.

Nice day for rememberin',
Stoppin' to think,
And startin'
Over again... It's a

> Nice day for a walk in the park,
> Easy lovin' day...

Richard Farquhar is an artist… a man who senses beauty, perceives and creates. To me, his name is Sandy. I was introduced to him by my partner, Frank. The two of them understand true friendship.

Sandy's deaf. He's hasn't always been deaf. When I first met him, he was an outgoing, active, healthy man in his late twenties. But Sandy, as I, was surprised. He also has an incurable disease. Sandy's disease is much more rare than MS. This particular disease caused him to lose his hearing.

When Frank first came to see me in February, he brought a letter from Sandy. I expected the old, "I know what you've been through," routine, but I didn't receive that treatment. I couldn't see well enough to read, so I asked Frank to read it for me:

Dear Bonnie,

I hope you are beginning to feel a little better by now. I have some idea of what you have been through and must be going through about now. It all gives more meaning to the old phrase, "payin' your dues." It's a lot easier to say, "Well, that's life", and let it go at that, when it's <u>someone else's</u> life. We can't shrug things off and adapt to new realities quite so easily when it's our own realities that are changing. But that's the problem.

After you get the physical demons under some kind of control (and, incidentally, the means of doing that in immunological diseases are increasing every day), then the next, and probably the biggest, problem is the mental one. Depression can be your worst enemy, but there are ways to lick that, too. Depression not only affects your outlook, your mood, what you do and you don't do; it can grind you down physically as well. It's a bad scene, but it's also the one you can possibly do the most about. (There are some drugs that can be helpful here, too.)

You soon learn to spot a pep talk or a hollow attempt to "cheer you up". You don't need them. You come to know what's possible and what isn't. You still need some tools for survival, though. One of them is to assess and accept the realities of your life. Then you need determination to make the most of the strengths and abilities that are left to you. These are greater than you imagine, but will take time and patience to discover. Don't be in a hurry. Keep your eyes and ears open.

Never give up. Never quit trying or believing in the possibilities of the future. Don't let anyone take over your life. It's still yours. You live it. Don't spend a lot of time looking backward. Sooner or later, your differences can become strengths as well as weaknesses. You will have some insights and understanding of things and yourself that are denied to most people. Don't be afraid to be different; learn from it.

Hang tough for a while and be patient. Things will start to come. There are many paths through the forest. There are far more possibilities than we are usually aware of. Look for them.

Don't indulge in the luxury of self pity. There's no help there, and there's no time for it. There's too much else that needs doing. Besides, you can always point to somebody else who is worse off and seems to be making it anyway.

Forget about what you always thought you <u>had</u> to do and what you thought your life <u>had</u> to be like. Do what you want to do and can do <u>now</u>. Spend some time finding out what that might be. Don't take pressure from anybody and don't put any on yourself.

Don't worry about money, either. Things have a way of working out. For one thing, you may be eligible for Social Security benefits in a few months. Check on it. Take everything you've got coming. It should include Medicare if you are eligible for disability benefits.

Sorry, I can't talk over the telephone. I would really like to hear from you. Drop a line if you feel like it, and stop by and see us next time you are up this way –

Later, Sandy"

The last page of his letter was an ink illustration, which he drew with a quotation by Menander: "We live, not as we wish to, but as we can."

I wish he could talk over the telephone… I wish he could hear…

Sandy continued to write to me. I appreciated his concern and his efforts to share his personal discoveries with me. Previously, our association had been through Frank. He had informed me of Sandy's progression, but I had avoided contacting Sandy personally. I had seen him a few times since his loss of hearing, but I felt very uncomfortable around him. And now, he was responding to the possibility of helping me. I felt so small…

I respect Richard Farquhar greatly. Each individual has experiences of his own, but there are physical and emotional reactions which seem common to all. Sandy's suggestions are universal:

"Dear Bonnie,

Got your letter today. It was really good to hear from you and learn that things are going a little better.

I hope you will write more letters, not just to me, but to everyone you would like to get in touch with. It is an old and excellent form of communication, even if it is less popular these days than yakking on the telephone. It is great therapy for the writer and often downright educational for the reader.

Many of your thoughts and feelings and some of your physical problems are familiar to me, too. When I lost my hearing, part of my natural balance was destroyed as well. Some of the early attacks left me dizzy and sick for days. The room would spin even when I was lying down. I would see double, lose my balance, fall and bump into things. Well, the inner ear damage which caused this has never completely been repaired, but, gradually, my eyes began to compensate and take over the function of maintaining my equilibrium. For a long time it was a great strain and caused much eye fatigue and incredible headaches. As time went on though, they became stronger and adapted to all the extra work and movement. Now, balance is no problem in normal situations, although in the dark (and in the water) I can't tell up from down.

Deafness is a big problem, and especially on top of everything else. I know many people are more uncomfortable about it than I am. I don't lip read everyone equally well, and it takes more time to "learn" some people's speech patterns than others, but if there's a pencil and paper handy, and a little time and relaxation, conversation goes fine, just a little slower.

The unpredictable ups and downs, the uncertainty, and the inconsistency in the way you feel in a disease like this is difficult to adjust to. Someone said you can get used to hanging if you hang long enough, but I'm almost certain whoever said it had never been hanged. As you said, it can be surprising how fragile our physical and emotional strengths seem to be and how quickly and completely they seem to crumble when the pressure is great enough. And yet, there is a resiliency about us, and reserves of strength and will, that we are unaware of until we need them. I'm a religious skeptic, too, but I can still recognize a strong force in us that demands and strives for life, regardless of the difficulty, usually.

Negative and morbid thinking seem to bottom out after awhile and turn upwards again. After you have faced the real possibility of death, accepted it, and even at your lowest points, desired it (and I have, too), then when you begin to look up again, you feel a new peace and freedom enter your mind. You are liberated, at least somewhat, from that fear in a way that many people perhaps are not.

I think it's helpful, for awhile anyway, to live a day at a time as it comes. Find some meaning and pleasure in it, even if in a small way, and be adaptable to the demands that come. Lie down and rest whenever you need to - once, twice, ten times a day. See people or don't, whatever you feel like. The future will gradually begin to shape up without much strain or conscious planning. You need time, more experience and experimenting to find out your needs, strengths, limitations- even if it all seems an impossibly slow and unpromising task. Still, things go better, and more possibilities become viable if you can keep the mental turmoil to a minimum.

Weakness and fatigue have been constant problems for me, too. I've found it pays to rest as much as I need to, not push myself beyond reasonable limits, and not worry or become frustrated over what I'm not getting done. But rather, I just try to enjoy the things I do work at and make the most of the times when I feel the best, then take it easy and try to be patient through the rough going whenever it comes. Also, don't hesitate to keep the doctors posted on just how you feel and what you need. If you can't sleep, get sleeping pills. If you're depressed or feeling like you're losing your mind, tell them and get some medication or at least advice. Don't be too much of a Spartan and make things any tougher than they have to be. There's an old saying, "there's no great loss without some small gain." In the case of problems like ours, one of the small gains is a good deal of insight and self knowledge that is denied to many. It's really good to think through to the bottom of a few things and to communicate to others about them. There's already enough nearly meaningless conversation in the world. Besides, I've learned that it is dangerous to bottle up your thoughts, fears, and emotions. It's like loading a bomb and you eventually explode.

Don't feel you have to "answer" these letters. Just write if and when you feel like it. I'll be glad to hear from you. Say hi to Bob.

Later,

Sandy

The last time I saw Sandy, his wife and he came to take me out to lunch. He was personally delivering a present to me, a handmade book which he had created. It was actually a lengthy poem called Corson's Inlet, written by A. R. Ammons and illustrated by Sandy. The inscription read, "Bonnie, I hope you find in here some pleasure and some rest for the mind. Sandy"

The book begins with, "I went for a walk over the dunes again this morning…" and continues to make observations of the inlet interwoven with the author's personal philosophy. The conclusion of the last page is, "that I have perceived nothing completely, that tomorrow a new walk is a new walk."

How beautiful! The world is always changing; each day is a new day… It has always amazed me how some people are articulate enough to express emotions which are common to many. It's nice to know that others share similar feelings.

I met Howard Lycett, an Episcopal minister, through Frank also. He would occasionally bring people from his parish into the clubs where we were performing to hear our group. This is not an ordinary practice associated with priests, checking out the Denver nightlife scene, but Father Hal is no ordinary priest… Wearing his white collar and his black pants and shirt, he's been known to even sample a drink in a bar! But, being more of a taster that a drinker, he's more interested in the music and the people who are present.

Recuperating from my MS attack, I responded to a knock at my mother's door one day to find Father Hal. He came in, sat down, questioned me about my condition and expressed his sympathy. He then began to optimistically explain his personal awareness of MS cases.

People who share the same illness are automatically classified and compared to others in their diseased group. The fact that so-in-so is doing well is apparently supposed to encourage you to do better. I never did understand the relationship between the two, how one individual case can be optimistically chosen to represent an entire group.

I wasn't in my best mood when Father Hal arrived but I did appreciate his effort and his time. Before leaving, he surprised me with a question: he asked if he could bless me now. Now, this was something new! Would I allow him to say a blessing for me! Why not...? Whether you are a religious believer, agnostic, or atheist, fear can make you search for anything to believe in. A psychology teacher of mine once said, "It doesn't matter what you believe in... as long as you believe in something."

I had never been asked if someone could say a blessing for me before, but I realized that I did need to depend on something. Father Hal put one hand on my head, made the sign of the cross with the other, and then offered a personal prayer for me. The seriousness of this short ceremony frightened me, but I was impressed, emotionally. Hal Lycett had outwardly offered a prayer specifically for me! Life can also be beautiful at times...

He then continued to speak of a friend of his who has MS, Patricia Peduzzi. Pat is a young woman in her late twenties who, like me, was surprised with the diagnosis, only she was less fortunate... She lost her sight. Pat is now completely blind because of this incurable disease. As with Sandy, they had each experienced the miraculous sense, which they later lost.

Pat is a rare example of strength. She continued her education with the help of special aids, and she is now teaching psychology. Her determination achieved accomplishment. Her story was impressive but not particularly inspirational to me. I admired this woman for her courage, but I realized that Pat was not me, and I was not her...

Several days later, I received a call from Father Hal telling me that he and Pat had stopped by my mother's house the day before, only to find me gone. I explained that a friend of mine had taken me out for lunch. He then asked if I would be available the following day for a visit from Pat and himself. My luncheon date had been a rarity; I would be home.

My first reaction to having missed them the day before, was relief. I wasn't encouraging visitors yet, and I was quite uncomfortable around other people, especially those whom I'd never met before. It seemed to me that Father Hal was rather eager to display his model success case of MS. My only previous experience with handicapped people had been in physical therapy at the hospital, and I wasn't anxious to be reminded of that time.

I imagined Pat to appear with all kinds of possible problems. Would she be able to hold her head up? I didn't know what other effects from the MS to expect. Would her eyes seem to focus or would they wander uncontrollably? Would her appearance be too much of a shock for me to emotionally handle? I wasn't anxious to meet her; I thought I'd be better off keeping my blessing and attempting my own personal success story.

But each day is a new day; I nervously awaited my visitors. Following their arrival, the most unusual sight in the room was me, chain-smoking Pat's cigarettes! She looked fine and appeared quite normal. She carried a cane which she later folded up. Her eyes gave no indication of her blindness. She was even able to look in the direction of the person she was speaking to . She actually made me feel quite comfortable. My smoking resulted from the nervousness of meeting anyone new at that time.

Father Hal had been right; I was immediately impressed with this woman. Her presence was calming; she spoke in a very composed manner and had an easy sense of humor.

She first asked me if it made me uncomfortable to be around handicapped people. I admitted that it did. She then suggested that I stay away from them. Uncomfortable feelings seem to be contagious.

She shared with me some of her experiences, her satisfactions, and her disappointments. The conversation never seemed forced; I received no lectures. We shared a relaxed interchange of MS experiences. It made me realize I wasn't alone…

Pat was a member of the Colorado MS Society. I was aware of its existence, but I had not contacted the agency. A personal friend of mine, who is a doctor, had called me earlier recommending that I should call the society. He provided a specific name and phone number for me to call. I called.

In 1974, there were three major societies dedicated to MS; The Rocky Mountain Center for Neurological Diseases, the National MS Society and the Colorado Society. The major purpose of the National Society was fund raising for research. The MS Society of Colorado was a United Way Agency that served patient needs throughout the state offering social activities and patient assistance programs, while promoting research.

When I called the society the first question I was asked was about my present condition. I now believe that I was a poor judge of my condition at that time… Who was I to judge? I realize that my society person had to determine a few things before beginning our conversation, but I was actually incapable of determining what my present condition was!

I answered with, "I'm feeling fine… now." Now, there was an indefinite reply if there ever was one! "Fine", compared to what? Compared to when I couldn't get out of bed; couldn't stand up straight, couldn't walk, or couldn't eat… I was feeling fine.

I also felt that mentally I had returned to normality, but, looking back, I now believe that I had not. With time, I thankfully continued to improve beyond my "feeling fine" stage.

My Society lady had no other choice than to believe that I was now "fine". Apparently, she was an advocate of a Low Fat Diet theory which was proposed by Dr. Roy L. Swank, Professor and Head of Neurology at the University of Oregon Medical School in Portland, Oregon. The diet supposedly reduced the number of attacks and their severity.

Now this was a change from the answers which I had received from Dr. Ginsburg. The society told me, "the diet has proven to be successful with those actually on the diet."

Was this possible? Could this be an answer for me, to reduce my attacks or make them less severe? She sounded so definite and convincing, offering me a possible treatment. She even gave me phone numbers of patients who were on the diet so that I could talk to them personally about their success. I immediately wondered why Dr. Ginsburg hadn't suggested this?

She continued to give me personal case histories to support her claims. One MS patient, who had been on the Low Fat Diet for 8 years could now "even play golf again!" I thought that case was a rather poor example of progress. Anyone who can swing their arms can play golf. Then, all you have to do is get back in the golf cart and ride to the next hole... I found little comfort in this case. She never did say how <u>well</u> she played golf...

Then there were other examples: someone had traveled all over the world and had been able to remain strictly on her diet, although she did have her problems with the cooks. Then, another lady was regaining her speech ability which had been disrupted.

My Society lady meant well. She tried to convince me of something in one phone conversation which the doctors had been unable to do. She gave me hope... She offered hope to arrest the progression of an incurable disease. My doctors had provided vague, indefinite answers, a game of wait and see. She had provided a definite course of action.

I was almost convinced. I intended to call the phone numbers given me. She had given me some hope, but she had also frightened me with her example cases. Maybe I expected too much. Maybe playing golf was a success. I'm sure, it must have been a success for that individual. Maybe it would be a success for me also. Only time would tell...

And time was the one thing the diet emphasized. The diet was supposed to begin as soon as possible after diagnosis of the disease. It became less effective the longer you waited. The Society even provided a registered dietitian for patient supervision and full understanding of the Low Fat Diet.

I asked two major questions to conclude my conversations: Is there any way to distinguish if improvement is caused by the diet or if it is just a result of the natural course of the disease, a remission? Does anyone on your staff actually have MS? The answer to each was no. There is no way to prove that the diet is responsible for improvement. But still, there is no way to prove that it is not. When there are so few choices and it involves your health, it never hurts to try suggestions, especially those that others believe in.

But hope is also a very powerful ingredient. I wondered if this could be a major connection with the diet program. If someone offers an answer, a definite plan, when others are still perplexed and confused, there is an instinct in each of us that directs us to try anything in an attempt to survive or regain normality. Could belief in a special program, a diet, give a person the needed mental and physical strength to challenge the disease? If you believe something will make you well, can it influence your improvement? The powers of the mind seem miraculous. Since my disease affects the brain and the nervous system, I would think that positive, optimistic thought could only be helpful. As with any disease, it doesn't ever hurt to try.

I am skeptical about special diets. As soon as people realize they have an incurable disease, they begin experimenting, trying to find a cure. Who else would be a more perfect test case? Special diets are easy enough to arrive at and then to follow up.

Everything from special exercise programs to meditation or strange religious cults is offered and encouraged by someone as a cure. Everyone's looking for the answers... You can always find articles such as "How I Cured MS" for almost any <u>incurable</u> disease. I wonder how doctors react to this material. I guess if I ate only apples for the rest of my life and the MS went into a long remission, I could say that apples cure MS, but there is still no way to determine that my remission wouldn't have occurred if I had not eaten the apples.

I am not presently on any special diet. I asked Dr. Ginsburg about the MS Low Fat Diet. He didn't encourage it, nor discourage it, but only said that it did not always prove to be helpful, so I decided that I'd try something like transcendental meditation and just forget the diet.

Anyway, the diet seemed to discourage eating all of the things which I liked. I wonder if they're trying to tell me something... No one really knows. I'm not on Dr. Swank's Low Fat Diet now... but I may live to regret it.

Today, MS organizations include The Heuga Center for Multiple Sclerosis which is now called Can Do Multiple Sclerosis, 1-800-367-3101, www.heuga.org), The Multiple Sclerosis Society of Colorado, and The National Multiple Sclerosis Society (NMSS), 1-800-344-4867, www.nmss.org. The National Society raises funds for research, serving the needs of MS patients to find the cause of the disease, alleviating symptoms, and providing information about Multiple Sclerosis. Relying on evidence based outcomes, the National Multiple Sclerosis Society and it's Colorado Chapters do not support any special diets today, and their staff does include MS patients.

Other organizations include The Rocky Mountain MS Center www.mscenter.org, www.uccc.info/conditions/brain-nerves/ms/ms-clinic@uch.aspx and the Multiple Sclerosis Alternative Healing and Wellness Center, www.msalternativehealingcenter.com

There are additional organizations, and I'm sure each one has their own success stories.

# <u>Love me, 'til the Rain Goes Away</u>

*You let the fire go low again, and I can feel the chill,*
*Now the rain is coming in, along the windowsill.*
*Won't you pour me one more glass of wine and tell me that you'll stay,*
*And love me... 'til the rain... goes away*

*I can't believe we found this place, so far from everywhere,*
*Where you could light a fire and I could dry my hair.*
*Won't you listen while I tell you things I've never tried to say,*
*And love me... 'til the rain... goes away*

*Just lay your head beside me now, and let me think of you,*
*As someone who could care for me, yet live without me too.*
*Won't you tell me that you'll stay with me, if only for today,*
*And love me... 'til the rain... goes away*

I was improving. My equilibrium was close to normal. I was riding my bicycle, with my sister, and my walking distance had lengthened. My vision had improved also. At least, it seemed to have leveled off a bit, although it still varied daily; some days still being better than others.

But then, for a few days in a row, things didn't look so good to me ... literally, my eyes seemed to be progressively getting worse. Everything seemed to be getting blurrier and I even noticed that the light didn't seem to be as bright as usual. In a self experiment, trying to determine my exact problem, I found it to be in my right eye. In the bathroom, I'd cover each eye separately with one hand, and then look into the mirror. I discovered that the vision in my right eye was very blurry and the light was very weak. I excused this as well as possibly deciding that the nerve must be experiencing some disturbance. Hopefully, I would regain its use in a day or two.

I was worried about it though. I told Bob that my eyes were bothering me and soon afterwards I became very interested in wearing sunglasses outside. There seemed to be more of a glare from the lights, both indoors and outside. With no assurance of improvement, I tried to cope with the blurriness.

Then, while reading a sentence, written on a piece of paper, I noticed that it just didn't seem to make any sense. I went back over it to find another word which I hadn't seen the first time. It just hadn't been there. The sentence was written on a white page and apparently the word had seemed white also. It appeared as a space, part of the page. This scared me... The doctor had told me in the hospital that I had blind spots in my vision, but this was the first time I had actually noticed it. I thought that my eyes had improved... that the blind spots were only temporary. Maybe my eyes were just tired... they needed to rest from too much strain. I went back to bed.

When I explained my experience to Bob, later that same day, he convinced me to call the doctor. Dr. Ginsburg has an answering service. Since I did need to set up another regular appointment anyway, I at least felt like I had an excuse to call.

I guess I didn't really need an excuse. He had always been so understanding with me; I just didn't want to bother him with my complaints. I'm sure that he had more important matters to deal with.

And anyway, what could he do? I had confidence in him… but I was far from impressed with the known treatments for MS.

I called the answering service and made my appointment. Then, I asked if they would give Dr. Ginsburg a message for me. Would they please tell him, "I can see very little out of my right eye." I didn't wish to talk to him; I just felt like I wanted him to be aware of any new developments.

Soon afterwards, the phone rang. It was the answering service. Dr. Ginsburg wanted to see me the next day.

It had been a week since my right eye began its digression. Dr. Ginsburg had seriously tried to impress me with the importance of calling him immediately whenever I noticed changes in my condition, so, at this new visit, trying to explain my hesitation to call, I expressed some doubt in doctors' ability to influence MS. I was then told that I was incapable of making the decisions, which were even difficult for him. I realized I had to depend on him… I couldn't argue about that.

When I arrived at the doctor's, we moved from our conference office to another room. I was seated on a table; Dr. Ginsburg turned off the lights. After shining a little flashlight in my eye for a while, the lights were back on and we moved on to the hallway where the eye chart was hanging.

I covered my right eye and read the letters at the end of the hall. Then I covered my good eye. Dr. Ginsburg asked me what the letter was; I couldn't see it. In fact, I couldn't even see the eye chart!

He was standing at the eye chart. He held his arms out and asked me to look straight ahead. He asked if I could see anything. It was blurry but I was aware of the movement of his arms. He then asked me to tell him how many fingers he was holding up as he walked toward me. By the time that he was two inches from my nose, I could see two fingers. Things didn't look so good, for me, or to me. Dr. Ginsburg prescribed prednisone. (I later learned that it is used to suppress the immune system or to decrease inflammation.)

I was vaguely familiar with this because of Pat. She had taken prednisone at one time for her eyes after she had gone blind. I remembered that she told me that it helped to restore some of her vision; some light and vagueness of impressions were visible but, unfortunately, this was only temporary for her.

I also remembered, she told me that she gained 30 pounds while on the medication! Now this was alarming to me! I'm one of those people who gains weight just by looking at food! Although I hate to admit it, my eating habits are not exemplary of a nutritionally balanced diet. I've always eaten what I felt like, when I felt like it.

But gaining weight does demand some personal eating restrictions, and being in the spotlight, entertaining, has a tendency to make weight gains very evident. Regardless of the possibilities of returning to my profession, the possibility of gaining 30 pounds horrified me! Going blind was one thing, but I didn't want to be fat. That's all I needed, more problems... At least, I was aware of the weight problem. So, I decided I just wouldn't eat while taking the medicine.

Dr. Ginsburg began writing out a prescription schedule for me to follow for the next twenty days. With four-day intervals, I was to take a decreasing number of these pills, with my meals. He drew a chart on a piece of paper designating the days and divided each day into breakfast, lunch and dinner. I was to begin by taking 12 pills a day; 4 with breakfast, 4 with lunch and 4 with dinner. It certainly sounded like a lot, but fortunately, they were small. Dr. Ginsburg emphasized the fact that I should take the medicine only with meals.

Now this was going to create a problem. It's difficult to stop eating, and take medication only with meals. I asked the doctor what constituted a breakfast and he answered, eggs, toast and juice. He sounded pretty serious about this eating business.

Breakfast, lunch and dinner... I hadn't eaten three regular meals a day since I was in Junior High School! And even then, I had to watch my weight. With a prescription like this, I'd end up looking like a blimp!

Then there were added directions. I was supposed to drink two large glasses of orange juice a day and take a tablespoon of Maalox 3 times daily in between meals. Possible side effects were explained and I was warned of irregularities to watch for: I was told that I may have some sleepless nights and also, prednisone could produce a state of euphoria.

The dictionary defines euphoria as "a feeling of great happiness

or well-being; bliss; ecstasy." The prednisone might make me high...
now this was more like it! I may be fat, but I'd be cheerful! I only
hoped that they'd give me something that would disguise any reality
of being overweight.

The size of the medication was no indication of its strength. The
pills were small, but they were powerful! Prednisone can be very
hard on the stomach; it can cause ulcers. I imagine that's why it was
important to have regular meals, to keep something in my stomach
all of the time. So it was eat, or have my stomach eaten up. Suddenly,
I became very interested in eating three meals a day...

I was more worried about the possibility of gaining weight, than
I was about the improvement of my eye. If I had to eat, my only
chance was to eat foods that weren't fattening. My mother-in-law
had a library of special diet books which covered everything from
alcoholic diets to eating your favorite foods, so I knew right where
to go to find the diet of my choice...my mother-in-law.

I decided to stick to the old-fashioned diet plan of counting
calories. My meals were planned (in the book), and I had my Maalox,
orange juice, and pills. I was ready to begin.

In the meantime, Dr. Ginsburg had set up a few more
appointments for me. I was supposed to see a doctor whose specialty
was "ophthalmology" or what is defined as "the medical specialty
encompassing the anatomy, functions, pathology and treatment of
the eye."

The next day I was scheduled to return to the hospital where I
had been, for another eye examination on their vision machine. I had
been through this same test, two times before. It didn't hurt, but it was
tiring. I'd just look in the machine, focus on the center light, and push
a buzzer whenever I was aware of a tiny moving light approaching
one of the sides.

So it was back to the hospital for me. Just the idea of returning
made me nervous. At least this time I would be able to sign in at the
desk, legibly.

After the hospital, it was the ophthalmologist's turn. He had
already received my vision charts from the day before. These are
diagrams which appear like a storm center on a weather map. A

number of circles in decreasing size are inside of each other. Then, there are numbers marking something and irregular lines marking the visual field. It looked like Greek to me! It was one of those secret doctor's messages which can only be understood after years of education...

After a few questions and a lot of looking, my new eye doctor recommended continuation of Dr. Ginsburg's prednisone schedule. I asked if he could determine if there was any permanent nerve damage to my eye. He told me that he couldn't tell yet; we would just have to wait. That sounded familiar.

Both he and Dr. Ginsburg tried to explain my eye condition to me, but the explanations were given at a time when I was nervous, and mentally, I was having trouble following them or concentrating. I appreciated their effort to inform me, but I left each office with only a vague understanding of my problem. I only knew that my present eye problem was different than the peripheral vision loss and the blind spot condition which I had experienced while I was in the hospital.

I now had, from my understanding, the same old inflammation of a nerve, the optic nerve, but the vision loss originated "in" the eye rather than being a misconnection between the brain and the eye. I have since learned that "the optic nerves connect to the retinas of the eyes with the brain," according to the American Heritage Dictionary of the English Language. Optic neuritis is an inflammation of the optic nerve, causing sudden blurriness in the eye which may progress in a few days, to temporary blindness and progressive loss of vision.

I could only distinguish forms of people with my right eye. Only individual's voices made them recognizable. I was told that generally these conditions improve, but my doctor couldn't determine if it definitely would, or how long improvement would take. So my vision might improve, possibly some, possibly none, and it might recur and cause loss of vision... No promises were made.

My eye doctor wanted to see me again in two weeks. Now, my sight would depend on some tiny little white pills called prednisone. So it was back to Maalox, orange juice and my pills.

Fear can destroy almost anything. The fear of blindness began with my realization that it could actually happen to me. It's always easy to be strong when we imagine ourselves adjusting to, or coping with, emergencies or personal loss. I always thought that I could handle it, but I believe that we continue not because of our emotional strength, but merely because we have to. I had no choice, no alternative. I wasn't strong… I was weak. My only choice was to use any strength that was available to me. I never knew how much I cherished the light of vision until it began to fade.

Darkness became my enemy. We have all closed our eyes, pretending to be blind, trying to experience how well we could do without the light. Through our sense of touch, we felt things and seemed to maneuver surprisingly well. But when the game was over, our blindfolds came off, our eyes opened, and the light returned.

Now all I could see was the light slowly leaving, not knowing if it would ever return. My game had no ending. I wasn't even interested in how clearly I could ever see again. Just some light, any light, meant everything!

It seemed to take a few days before I noticed any visible change. Then the slow improvement began with my awareness of more light.

The following weeks were a combination of planning my diet meals, refilling my prescription bottle, and drinking cans of orange juice and bottles of Maalox. Each day I would cover my good eye to see what I could see.

My major improvement occurred during the first week when the medication dosage was the highest. I was still unable to actually distinguish anything. But, at least I was now aware when something was there. Outlines and images became apparent although they appeared dim and extremely blurry. I still couldn't see well enough to recognize anyone with only my right eye. But I was thankful… the light had brightened.

I returned to see Dr. Ginsburg about two weeks after my prednisone prescription. I got the same old lights in the eyes and counting the fingers treatment. This time, I could guess that there were two fingers up at a distance of about four feet away, but I still couldn't read the largest print on the eye chart.

Dr. Ginsburg said that he couldn't see much improvement in my vision, but that I was definitely walking better. I didn't particularly agree with him. I could tell a great deal of improvement in my vision and hadn't noticed much change in my leg. Whenever I became excited or nervous, my leg would become weak and shaky. This varied throughout the day. I explained this to him.

Evidently, he was happy to see me walking better at that particular moment. He said that the improvement was noticeable to him, that I may have forgotten what I was like when I was in the hospital.

Now I <u>was</u> beginning to worry. Maybe he'd forgotten! Was he confusing me with another patient? I felt if anyone should remember, it should be me! But then again, my memory had not been working well lately. I was only satisfied that he recognized some improvement, anywhere!

Although I continued to take the prednisone, my condition had seemed to level off. At least I couldn't see any more visible improvement. If the eye was improving, the progress was too slow to be recognized immediately.

One thing, which I was proud of, I hadn't gained any weight yet. In fact, I hadn't even noticed any increase in my desire to eat. With my lack of self-discipline, I was thankful for that.

And, as far as I knew, I didn't have any signs of ulcers. At least, I didn't have any stomach pain or aching. The prednisone didn't seem so bad, as long as it was accompanied by my diet plan.

Then, on the other hand, "not so bad" is a matter of judgment. It wasn't that great either! Unfortunately, the one side effect I had been counting on seemed to be nonexistent in my case. Where was my euphoric state? I certainly hadn't noticed any rush of ecstasy…

But I did notice the nervousness which accompanied my little white pills. Loud noises almost scared me to death and even quieter ones affected me. The prednisone made me feel "jittery" nervous, high-strung, and irritable. So the fact that the medication didn't seem so bad to me doesn't necessarily mean that others around me would agree that it affected them in the same way.

<u>They</u> had to adjust to <u>my</u> temperament. There were periods of time when I was incapable of getting along with anyone, including myself. Other people only frustrated and irritated me. Differences of opinion between individuals seemed unresolved, agreements impossible.

My disease certainly seemed contagious in some respects. The emotional pressures, which had been concealed, were now erupting.

I believe in the transmission of energy vibrations between people and the possible detection of good feelings by what has been termed "good vibrations". Hiding emotions was impossible at the time. And, tension doesn't allow for "good vibrations".

I realized that my little white pills were responsible for my disagreeable moods, and I realized that I was responsible for the emotional eruption. The medication was definitely affecting my personal strength to conceal my emotions. I was indifferent to others attitudes and selfishly felt as if it was their problem, not mine, to be able to cope with me. I felt entitled to release my tensions which were mounting.

The realization of my disease was now becoming more of a reality to me. I HAVE MULTIPLE SCLEROSIS. And yet, I never did ask, "Why me?" I guess I never felt worthy of questioning. I was only grateful that, if someone had to get an incurable disease, it had been me rather than someone whom I loved. I think that I would have suffered more, worrying about another, than I did by actually experiencing the disease myself.

Only I am aware of my emotional state, my pain, my worries, my discomfort. Others may be informed, but only I will ever actually know for sure. It is my lone secret. Even if I try to reject the secret, if I desire to inform others of my experiences and my thoughts, I am still limited by language and my personal ability to explain. I am dependent on communicating feelings and emotions with a group of words whose definitions even vary. Maybe everyone is restricted purposefully. Maybe each of our secrets was individually designed for us.

I think that it is impossible to realize just how restricted we are in communication until we experience something which is uncommon, and then try to relate our feelings to others. I felt isolated. In this isolation, I began to seek someone or something to share my experiences with. At this point, it was only natural for me to go beyond reality, looking for a god, a creator. And, for some reason, there was a comforting feeling in this association.

I experienced a kind of closeness to nothingness... Nothingness, in the sense that there was not a specific form but there seemed to be a feeling of space. I experienced a feeling of suspended peacefulness. I felt as if I were supported by buoyancy in a void.

My association was less of a physical identification, and more of an inner feeling. I felt secure... I think I can best describe this with a dictionary definition: "secure: 1. Free from danger or risk of loss; safe. 2.free from fear or doubt; not anxious or unsure." I felt confident in something and at peace with myself.

Illness gave me an awareness of the human communication gap. Our personal experiences are ours alone. I realized and feared isolation and looked for something that would provide security and peacefulness. Other worldly things became insignificant. I was selfishly "on my own trip", I recognized my selfishness but felt that this state would eventually come to each of us. There's no way for me to explain it. I only seemed to fade away and become unconcerned about others.

MS is a disease of the central nervous system. Since the central nervous system is the brain and the spinal cord, there is a visible, physical change in the brain itself, which may be accompanied by mental changes. Regardless of the disease, I would assume that the medication and drugs which are used could have a similar effect. My disease isolation stills occurs and I don't think that I'm that unique.

Most of us have felt the pain and loss of having someone who is close to us die. I still remember my grandmother, as she lay in the hospital bed, her eyes closed, as if she was in a coma. I wondered if she was aware of my presence. I wondered if she could even hear me. Why didn't she respond? I only wanted some indication of her awareness.

But there was none... I left the hospital, frustrated, not understanding.

I guess I'll never know, but I experienced a mental state which I believe may have been very similar to hers. Possibly, she was on "her own trip". Maybe she was on a trip which is intended for each of us... a trip which may explain our creation and cause us to be indifferent to our physical, living state. This isolation stage may be a needed preparation for the change toward accepting the unknown.

My disease has given me a strength; I am liberated from a fear. I no longer fear death. Fear, personal loss, sorrow, is for the living... not the dead. My journey into the unknown was not fearful, it was comforting and reassuring. For me, there seemed to be no awareness of time or place, and no concern for others that I was leaving behind. There was only a peaceful acceptance.

Being an agnostic, I emerged from my experience as a believer in something. My belief didn't come into being from my acceptance of having an incurable disease and my search for help to survive. My belief came out of my mental trip. It developed from a feeling... a feeling that caused me to believe in something.

My something is a creator, an indefinable force... "my god". It can direct my thoughts and calm my fears. It controls me. It has the power of life. Whatever it is, it seems to handle things for me.

I still don't go to church, and I still continue to question reasons for my existence. I have no answers to offer to anyone. I only know that I have gained confidence in something that directs me and a realization of my weaknesses and my inabilities.

After my MS attack, Frank told me that he envied me. At the time, when I received this astonishing information, I was confused and discouraged. I felt that Frank was equally as confused! He explained that he envied me because I would gain experiences which others could not. I now understand. "There's no great loss without some small gain."

I was on no medication at the time that my religious trip occurred. MS does affect the brain. ACTH can also cause disorientation. Whether my thinking was rational or irrational, makes no difference to me. The fact that I was made comfortable because of it, does.

After the prednisone, it was time to go back to my opthalmologist again. The day before my appointment, I was surprised with a call from Dr. Ginsburg. Now this was a first... a doctor calling me! He asked about my eye and then went into reassuring claims supporting the ophthalmologist. I learned that the eye specialist was Dr. Ginsburg's personal doctor whom he had all the confidence in the world in.

I hung up the phone feeling that the call was very considerate of Dr. Ginsburg. It made me feel as though he was interested in my condition and that he highly respected my eye doctor. The reason for his call became evident the next day.

Sitting in the ophthalmologist's office, I remembered where we had left off the last time concerning my eye condition. If the prednisone didn't offer the proper treatment for my eye, he said he would have to "treat it". Now this leaves a great deal open to the imagination. I understood this to mean more medication. What else could they do to my eye?

After the examination, my ophthalmologist said that he was satisfied with the eye's progress and I wouldn't need the cortisone. After making him aware that I was ignorant of the cortisone treatment that he was referring to, I was informed. His reference to "treating" my eye referred to a shot of cortisone directly into the eyeball! If I had known that I might receive a shot into my eye, I wouldn't have slept for days, worrying about it. Needless to say, I was thrilled with the prednisone results and satisfied with my ignorance of eye treatments. Thankfully, I had avoided both the worry and the shot… at least this time.

# The Two Peddler Men

Many years ago
I swore that I would pen
The story of the market place
And the two old peddler men

As just a lad of twelve
I sat with them for hours
As one sold all discarded junk
while the other peddled flowers

(Refrain) Hey rich man
    (I got junk for sale)
    hey wealthy man
    (I got junk for sale)
    I've got flowers for your lady

    Hey rich man
    (I got junk for sale)
    hey wealthy man
    (I got junk for sale)
    Flowers, for your lady
    (Here's a pretty copper bucket)

And I marvel now
Even as I marveled then
To the story that was told
By those two old peddler men

For they seemed to say
That what we sell is ours
And I'm as proud to sell my junk
As he to sell his flowers

(Refrain)
Well the market place is gone now
But the two old men are not
For they are part of those of us
Content with what we've got.

And I believe
We'd all be better then,
If everyone could listen to
Those two old peddler men.

# V

## Fifth Month

## March

I was constantly looking for some sign of visible progress. When some improvement was obvious, it would then stop or even regress back to an earlier stage or poorer condition. This made me feel as if I had achieved my nearest to normal stage. I expected my progress to either continue or to completely stop. I wasn't familiar with such an erratic pattern of progression and remission which is characteristic of MS.

Patience can only be suggested, it cannot be taught. Hopefully it can be learned, or at least accepted more easily with time. Patience and optimism may be the only defense against depression. For me, depression was unavoidable. I can only suggest for others to expect the worst and prepare their optimistic defense early. Then, support your defense, even during the times when optimism seems impossible... especially during the times when it seems impossible.

Some improvement seemed to continue both physically and mentally. I decided that if exercise was beneficial for physical improvement, then some problem solving might be helpful mentally. And, it just so happened that I had some mathematical problems to solve before April 15th.

This is the recognizable time of the year when taxes are due. Being a professional entertainer, I am considered to be self-employed. Self-employment means that nothing is automatically deducted from your monthly pay. You're supposed to pay the quarterly estimate, the amount depending on your previous year's earnings, but if it's more convenient for a self-employed individual to pay his taxes according to a yearly estimate rather than quarterly, this is also acceptable.

This year, I had paid nothing to the government so far, and I was depending on my contracts through March to cover my income taxes for the year... What's that old saying? "Don't count your chickens before they hatch." Well, my chickens never hatched and besides that, they caught a disease, and couldn't even lay eggs!

It's not unusual for people who are self-employed to depend on an expected income, which is verified by something as definite as a legal contract. You just don't expect to get sick or injured! At least, I didn't. The only time that I had missed a night performing for the last five years, was once, due to losing my voice. When you entertain, you perform and smile... sick or well. "The show must go on!"

My mental exercise game began with organizing my bills and figuring personal deductions. Frank was actually in charge of issuing our checks, financing group loans and accounting for group expenses. He was our business manager, but personal deductions were each members' own responsibility. This included such things as travel expenses, food, motel, personal loans, our mileage, show clothes, musical equipment and supplies, and album loss or profit.

For those people who are organized, this would be a minimal task. With my organization skills, this would have been a challenge under normal health conditions. Fortunately, I had enough time to correct my errors.

My income tax work only further confirmed my mental confusion. Some days I was better than others. Again, my condition constantly fluctuated from near normal decision power to what seemed to be insurmountable, confusing problems.

After a while, I was able to recognize the days when I wasn't as coherent as usual. On those days I didn't have much of a choice. It became impossible to complete what I had intended. Left without a choice, acceptance was my only answer. Both acceptance and waiting without answers, seemed to be unavoidable with my new disease.

Neither playing cards, nor chess, seemed to work well for my mental exercise program. I was never proficient in either, but I've always enjoyed them both, but now, remembering particular cards which had been played, or a chess strategy was impossible. My mind would be mentally clear one minute, allowing for decisions, and completely blank the next minute, having forgotten my plan. This was a definite competitive disadvantage. My opponents were aware of my condition and jokingly accepted my mental in-capabilities. Playing cards with relatives was a possibility, but I wasn't interested in entering a bridge tournament.

# <u>Stick It</u>

*Drivin' in traffic used to be a bore,*
*But it isn't that way, anymore.*
*Not with bumper stickers to read,*
*I've even cut down on my drivin' speed.*

*One kind's got gummy stuff on the back.*
*The other's the kind where you lick it.*
*Pick a spot on your bumper everyone can see,*
*Then get your sticker and stick it... pick it!*

*America the Beautiful,...Love it or leave,*
*Honk if you love Jesus, if you really do believe.*
*Save our environment, do it at any cost.*
*That was a tough little sucker to read,*
*It was covered with exhaust!*

*Don't you do it in the lake, don't you Californicate.*
*Do your part and pitch in. God loves you even if you sin.*

*Don't you think your philosophy should be (should be)*
*Somethin' everybody can see (can see)*
*And our country's doin' so darn well*
*Since everybody went to show and tell*

*Stick... your philosophy... (come on children)*
*Stick... your philosophy, (everybody) stick your philosophy,*
*I said... stick it! On the bumper of your car!*

# VI

## Sixth Month

## April

Although I was still unable to drive, I was concerned about the procedure to validate my license. I now optimistically expected improvement. The prednisone had at least helped my leg; my limping now occurred only occasionally. My right hand and arm seemed to be almost normal again. Now, my eyes were my major problem. My right eye was extremely poor and I still experienced vision variation in my good left eye. With both eyes together, I had no depth perception, quite a bit of blurriness, and a peripheral vision loss. Five months had passed since my attack. I called the driver's license bureau.

There seems to be a law for everything. The only confusion is finding out which law applies to what! I was now in the position of having what appeared to be a legal Colorado Operator's License while I was physically unable to operate a car. Well, that may not be entirely true... I could probably operate a car, but my reflexes left a lot to be desired. Both physically and mentally, I still wasn't responding very well. I still limped some at times, and my mental acuteness varied throughout the day.

Since driving a car demands alertness, proper vision, quick reactions, and the use of the right foot to accelerate and stop the vehicle, I definitely believe that my driving was impaired. I explained on the phone that I had recently been diagnosed as having Multiple Sclerosis, and I wanted to know what I should do to make my license valid.

Their major question was, "Has your license expired?" Since it had not, I was informed my license was valid. I then explained that my vision was very poor and asked if an eye test would be required. (It's difficult to drive safely when you can't see.) The officer at the bureau explained that my license was valid unless it had expired, and legally nothing could be required of me until my next license examination time. If I would like to come down and take an eye test, I was welcome to do that. And, if I got in an accident, my driving capabilities would then be tested.

For an optimistic view of an incurable disease, this guy was definitely encouraging. He was basically telling me that legally, I was "OK", valid, acceptable on the streets, until I got in an accident. There was no law restricting me from driving. Beyond legality, whether I drove or not was my decision.

I had expected a shocked reaction to my disease... or at least a required stamp on my driver's license, indicating my health condition. I got neither. My disease was accepted. I needed no health identification.

I not only felt incapable of driving, but also incapable of handling the responsibility of my decisions. It seemed to me that anyone with a disease which affects the brain, or anyone who is taking medication, should be restricted in some manner.

At the same time, I also realized that my impatient desire to improve would encourage me to continue to test myself. If I could drive legally, I would drive as soon as I felt confident. But who was I to judge my competence?

To judge indicates the necessity of testing. Testing then indicates what is possible, and the limits of possibility can only be established after determining what is not possible.

To determine my driving competence, I would first need to drive and then I'd discover my limitations. My driving might not only endanger myself, but it could also be unsafe for others to be on the streets. Human lives are a high stake... just to determine driving competence. It seems to me that when you need restrictions, there are none demanded, but when you don't need them, there's a law for everything... well, almost everything.

So it was my decision... Due to the financial investment which Allstate Insurance Company shares with me, I concluded that their office, rather than the license bureau, might be the restricting force on my future traveling. I didn't think that they could legally restrict me from driving, but a raise in my insurance rates could financially prevent me from returning to the highway.

So, my next step was to call the insurance company. Again, I was surprised. My insurance was fine; I needed no disease identification and there was no rate increase.

This was too good to be true! I couldn't believe it! How could there be such little concern, at a government bureau which examines individuals to issue licenses, to insure knowledge of driving regulations and laws? Why didn't my insurance rates go sky high?

My husband explained their disinterest. If I caused an accident or injury to someone else, I possibly could be sued. I'm not familiar with a case such as this, but I'm sure the legal ramifications could be lengthy, causing much discussion and confusion. It certainly made me question if driving was worth the consequences which could result.

Fortunately, my improvement continued to keep pace with my impatience, which, unfortunately, still continued. It had been almost seven months since I had last driven, before I went to Olympia, but I could legally drive and I wanted to.

I had been "without wheels" for some time, during which time I had experienced some amazing physical and psychological changes. I was anxious to drive, but I was also "scared to death!" It seemed as if it had been years since the last time that I had controlled a car. I desired the freedom which it offered. I only hoped that the fear which had developed would diminish with patience, time and practice.

- I began my relearning process by moving the car from the street into the driveway at my mother's home. I was attempting to get the feel of the car again, trying to remember where the gears were located and trying to differentiate distances to allow for my vision deficiencies.

There seemed to be a clear division between my potential and the machine. Each maneuver I did had to be thought through thoroughly before being initiated. Very little seemed to come to me merely as an automatic, unconscious response. After driving for ten years, my last seven months off had made an amazing difference. My relearning process reminded me of the severity of my mental problems and changes which were occurring.

After mastering the gear changes and trying to avoid the grass and bushes beside the driveway, I ventured out onto the street, intending to go around the block once. Now this was a bit different from my driveway driving! The driveway was mine alone, while the street was shared with other cars.

My mother's house is in a nice, quiet, suburban area where there's not a lot of traffic. In fact, on this first day out on the streets, I didn't even meet another moving vehicle on the whole block! But there were quite a few cars parked on the sides of the street. Trying to avoid these, I found the center of the street and, barely moving, I slowly inched forward.

On the left side of the car, I could see fairly well, accept for some blurriness. On the right side of the car, I couldn't differentiate distances to determine how close I was to anything! So I stuck to the center of the road, trying to analyze my new visual perspective. At least, I wasn't speeding!

Visual analysis takes concentration, so I held my top speed down for the day to a racy 10 m.p.h. But, at that time, it seemed like I was racing. The car seemed so big, so awkward and so uncomfortable. Any movement at all seemed faster than I could handle. Fortunately, I never met another car and I wasn't asked to move over, out of my center lane, so my "round the block trip" was completed successfully, without an accident. I returned my car back to its proper space on the street. A new challenge had been met… and my license was still valid.

## *Freeway, Flower Power, Petal Pusher*

*I was drivin' home, just the other day,*
*When I seen this lady, standin' by the freeway.*
*She was holdin' flowers,*
*While the cars kept movin' by*

*Well I pulled my truck to the side of the road,*
*I put her in reverse, and backed up real slow,*
*And said, "Excuse me, ma'am,*
*Do you need a ride?"*
    *She was a freeway, flower power petal pusher.*
    *A genuine concrete city, flower child*
    *Holdin' them flowers high, way up in the sky,*
    *Come on, buy a flower for your lady, make her smile...*

*Well, I pulled my car up to the light,*
*My radio was palyin', I was feelin' all right,*
*When I seen this guy, standin' on the corner,*
*Flowers stickin' out of his van,*

*The light was red, so I jumped out,*
*Got a dozen for a dollar, and when I turned around,*
*The light was green, and people were startin'*
*To make funny signs with their hands...*
    *(Chorus)*
*Now everybody wants to be his own boss,*
*If you're sittin' on the corner, with flowers all around your feet...*
*It don't pay much, but you're pretty free. Organic gardening's the word for me,*
*I bring a little piece of nature, right into the city streets...*
    *(Chorus)*

## *"Hank's Raisin' Hell in Heaven"*

*©2005 Bonnie Lynne Ellison / All Rights Reserved*

*His Mama played piano. He sang in the choir.*
*Alabama country folk, couldn't get much higher.*
*(he wrote) Coun-try classics, a Grand Ole' Opry star,*
*And died in his '53 Cadillac car...*

> *Hank's raisin' Hell in Heaven, He's raisin' Hell in Heaven, He's raisin' Hell in Heaven... Celebratin' Peace!*
> *He's got a party goin' on, He's got a party goin' on, He's got a party goin' on....That will never cease...*
> *Everbody's welcome...The good times never end,*
> *Hank's raisin' Hell in Heaven...with all his good old friends...*

*He can't stop smi'lin', he's out of control!*
*Endless "Happy hours", puts rhythm in his soul.*
*He's dan-cin' on the tables, sing-in' from raf-ters,*
*No more cheat-in' hearts, just love and laugh-ter.*
> *(chorus)*
>> *He was-n't perfect...without any sin,*
>> *But after Final Judgement, S-a-i-n-t P-e-t-e-r slipped him in...*
> *(music)*
> *(chorus) Amen*

# VII
## Seventh Month
## May

My next travel experience came shortly after my first trip. It was registered for future generations in my diary on May 28.

My diary reads: "First day that I drove more than a block, mailed American Song Festival tapes, put top down (on the car), felt a bit faint at the post office- wondered about the heat."

The "first day I drove" was underlined intentionally. I had conquered my own fear. Whether a challenge had been a wise decision was questionable, but I had succeeded. It may have been less than safe, but it certainly was good for my morale. It offered me a new sense of freedom and newly found self-confidence.

I probably wouldn't have driven if I hadn't had a special reason encouraging me. I had entered a songwriting contest, the American Song Festival. It is an international songwriting competition seeking new talent in the musical field. The contest seemed reputable, advertising in Billboard (a popular music trade magazine), newspapers, and it was supported by top entertainers in the field.

I'd already paid my entry fee, filled out my entry form and mailed it in. I then received a cassette tape to record the two entries of my original songs. Jerry offered his time and talent to contribute to my effort. He not only supplied his musical ability in accompanying me, but also offered to let me use his tape recorder.

The songs which I entered in the contest were my own, original material, but they had not been written recently. I had written them prior to my MS attack, prior to my mental confusion. I feared that I would never regain the gift of writing again. But, I did have confidence in the songs I chose to enter.

I really wasn't concerned with the reputability of the contest or even my chances of winning a portion of the cash prizes that were offered. I was concerned about becoming disassociated with the profession that I loved. I now felt unable to continue performing with the group and I didn't feel confident enough to do a single act. Outwardly, I generally appeared healthy; inwardly, the disease continued working in my mind. I seemed only to know what I couldn't do. I couldn't perform and I couldn't write songs of any quality.

But, as I learned from my muscles, exercising is important before their use is regained. Everything indicated to me that I should forget music, avoid the tense situations, but I felt like I was part of music, or it was a part of me so, rather than giving up, I decided to "exercise" my musical ability.

I wanted to do something… anything associated with music. I listened to it. I played what I could on my guitar, when my arm and fingers allowed me. I followed Billboard and even studied to increase my knowledge of the music business. And, now I was entering two of my own songs into the American Song Festival. The contest offered me a reason to continue with my music. It offered me a chance to be involved, even though my involvement was only through the mail…

Contests all have deadlines for entries. My contest tape was due, and the tape deserved some special type of recognition. I wished to send it by certified mail. At least I would receive someone's signature verifying OK delivery. So, I needed to go to the post office. I couldn't think of a better way to show my appreciation for the contest's encouragement than by my taking the tape myself, on my first real trial drive.

OK! The tape was mailed for $1.30 and I was on my way to becoming a real "star of tomorrow!" But I was fortunate. I didn't need to wait until tomorrow. Completing the contest and driving to the post office made me feel like a "star of today…"

Yes, I made it to the post office, but I felt a bit light-headed, as if I might faint. Although I've never fainted before, I thought that this might be a first. It wasn't a very encouraging sign to build up my confidence, since I hadn't driven in over half a year.

I had put the top down on my convertible, not for an ego trip and not trying to establish a new image of myself in my diseased condition, but for a more practical reason... my vision. I not only put the top down but I rolled all of the windows down also. I wanted nothing to interfere with my line of vision, especially because my line had been cut pretty thin already.

It was hot. The air felt good in the convertible, but the sun was trying to bake me alive! At least, it seemed to be trying to cook my brain in the five minutes it took to get to the post office.

My eyes seemed to be affected, being blurrier than usual, and my head felt light. Fortunately, these symptoms occurred after I was parked. I felt a lot safer, not moving. I shook my head a couple of times, trying to clear my vision. I even considered putting the top up on the car which is a sacrifice for a nature lover like myself. I finally decided to go into the air conditioned post office and leave my beloved sun outside. I left the top down.

After recuperating a few minutes inside, my tape package was stamped "certified mail" and disappeared behind the counter in preparation for its flight to Los Angeles.

I had made it to the post office, so I thought I'd try a new challenge, a twenty minute endurance drive. I still felt good. I could make it! I'd just go slow...

Twenty minutes gives anyone plenty of time for thinking. I found my mind was wandering rather than concentrating on driving or protecting me while I was on the road. I was just cruising along, thinking, but this was exactly what I was trying to avoid... thinking. In my condition, I certainly realized the necessity of being alert and conscious of my actions. Realizing this, I kept trying to redirect my attention toward driving. But my attention span was short. I could only seem to concentrate on driving for a minute or less and then I'd find myself drifting off again, paying no attention to the concentrated effort I needed to drive. I couldn't focus.

Then, I recognized something, which I could relate to... a hitchhiker. This was not only a hitchhiker, but a "male" hitchhiker. Since he had caught my attention and rekindled memories of my not so distant long-haired, hippie, "peace" days, I decided that his company might keep me away from the mental drifting that I was experiencing.

There he was, with his long hair and jeans, thumbing a ride down the road. There I was, on my first long distance trial drive (with an incurable disease) stopping to offer him a ride.

This wasn't a particularly new or unusual situation for me. Amid all the reports of the dangers of hitchhikers, burglaries, rapes and murders, I have been one of those people who almost seem to ask for trouble, and still have fortunately missed it. Anyway, with hitchhikers, I've always felt that the person doing the hitchhiking is far more vulnerable than the person who offers the transportation. I know that can be argued, but this day, almost unconsciously, without fear, I stopped.

We didn't talk much. He didn't need to go very far. His main desire at that time was to get to the interstate highway and to continue safely on his way. Not until he was in the car and we were driving along did I realize what I had done.

I, the one who had been so conscious of the possibility of an accident and the possibility of being wrongly accused because of the variation customary to my disease, was including an innocent hitchhiker in a situation that he was totally unaware of. I, who couldn't see to begin with, was possibly endangering this man's life. I was just the kind of help that this guy didn't need! If only he knew who he was riding with… If only he were aware of the quiet chance he was taking…

But he didn't need to go far. We soon stopped, he thanked me, and his thumb went up again, in a new direction. I'm sure that I wasn't the first chance he'd taken confronting danger… and I'm sure I wasn't his last.

## _Watermelon is a King's Delight_

_When I was just a small boy,_
_I never could grow old._
_Even when it snowed outside,_
_There wasn't any cold._

_I could love a river, or a robin, or a flower,_
_Or a cricket, chirpin' in the night._
_All of God's creation was mine to tell about,_
_Watermelon was a king's delight._

_When I was just a small boy,_
_Trees were nightly towers._
_I could watch an icicle_
_Or water, drip for hours._

_Wish I was an Indian, or a soldier or a cowboy._
_All the world would know my name._
_Stars were a mystery, dogs were a friend,_
_Little girls were very tricky game._

_Now I am a grown boy, not a soldier, not a cowboy._
_All the world don't know my name._
_Stars are still a mystery, dogs are still a friend,_
_Little girls are very tricky game._

_Age is not important, the heart remains a boy._
_Every day brings murmurings of another day of joy._

_I can love a river, or a robin, or a flower,_
_Or a cricket chirpin' in the night._
_All of God's creation is mine to tell about,_
_Watermelon is a king's delight._

Later that day, I drove over to a friend's home, a former entertainment partner of mine, Ralph Achilles. Ralph had originally performed with my partner, Frank, calling the duo Achilles and Frank. They had first tasted stardom with the popularity of their record, The Two Peddler Men, which Achilles wrote. Following their record, they toured throughout the United States and overseas, internationally!

Thinking back over the past years, I vividly remember the circumstances that brought us together. Everything looked good for the duo's entertainment career when Achilles received a friendly letter from Washington, D.C. It seems that Achilles had avoided his active military duty by enlisting in the reserves. Now his Selective Service System was notifying him that his country needed him.

The feeling was not mutual... the country may have needed the entertainer, but the entertainer wasn't particularly interested in defending his country at that particular time in his entertainment career.

But excuses can go only so far... Achilles was on his way to California, not to record, or to talk to agents or promoters, but to discover a fort, Fort Irving, the army's Mojave Desert post, located between Los Angeles and Las Vegas, in the middle of nothing but sand, baked by the California desert sun. The entertainer, musician, songwriter was instantly transformed into an army man, defending you, me, and our country.

Having lost his partner, Frank meanwhile went back to Colorado State University in Fort Collins to work on his Master's degree. I was attending C.S.U. at the same time, trying to get through my junior year while singing as a single at a local 3.2 beer establishment. I sang downstairs, with no admission charge, just me, my guitar, and the bar.

Achilles and Frank had been there. Only, they had performed upstairs, with an admission charge. They had a one night booking, performing as they traveled through town.

I was going to school, when to my surprise, I found Frank in one of my American Literature classes, and I was further surprised when he told me that Achilles and he were considering adding a female to their group. He asked if I was interested.

I then got the story about Achilles being temporarily occupied, typing at Fort Irving, and how Frank and I could start entertaining as a duo. It would be transformed into a trio as soon as Achilles got out of the service.

I was impressed with Frank's offer. I stopped school, with the intention of returning after a year or two of "outside" experience.

Using our names as each group originated, Frank and Bonnie performed for one year together, followed by Frank, Achilles, and Bonnie (The F.A.B. Company), which was together for the next four years. Achilles then became interested in performing as a single, which he had done while he was in the army, so we all peacefully separated. Achilles went off to do his single, Frank and I continued together and added a musician, Jerry Jacobs, still calling ourselves The F.A.B. Company with Jerry Jacobs. This time, the F.A.B. Company initials stood for Frank And Bonnie. We had performed together for about one year when we arrived in Olympia, Washington. After my attack, Frank and Jerry continued entertaining as a duo, and Achilles remained as a single, only adding accompanists.

Unfortunately, personal discoveries are merely that... personal discoveries. Sometimes, they can't be applied universally. Each of us must find our own understanding.

I felt unable to express my experiences. "I don't know how to tell you where I've been." Even if I were able to, I felt that any serious attempt at writing would have to be in poetic form rather than being written as a song. So, I went to the opposite extreme.

I wanted to write material that avoided confusion or multiple personal interpretations. I wanted to write something direct, general, basic, commonplace or even what might be considered "trite", so I decided to try country. I'd try to write commercially acceptable country music.

My closest association with country music was the fact that I played the guitar. Well, that may not be entirely true... I did play the guitar, but I also was familiar with country life.

There may not be too many cowgirls who grow up in Baltimore,

Maryland and then move to Littleton, Colorado, but this one did. I moved to Colorado, rodeo-ed and heard plenty of country music while currying horses and shoveling stalls at the barn. I had been around country music, but I had never been very interested in it before. (The cowboys were much more interesting.) Our entertainment group would have been considered more "folk oriented", although we sang a variety of music. We were a show group, interspersing our music with comedy. The country material that we did was generally a spoof on country music. But now, I was approaching this music in a new light. Now I wanted to write "serious country."

# FAB COMPANY

SPECIAL THANKS TO DOUG OLSON ON DRUMS, MARVIN PERKINS ON BASS
AND RICK McCOLLISTER ON PIANO.
PRODUCED BY : FRANK BRUEN, JERRY JACOBS & RICK McCOLLISTER
ENGINEER: RICK McCOLLISTER
A&R: GREEN DANIEL
PHOTOGRAPHY: STEVE FRINK
COVER CONCEPT, DESIGN AND PRODUCTION: MEDIA GRAPHICS
SPECIAL THANKS TO MARCIA SPURLOCK FOR HER HELP AND MORAL SUPPORT
RECORDED AT APPLEWOOD STUDIOS, GOLDEN COLORADO

**SIDE ONE**

1. EASY LOVIN' DAY
   B. Ellison
2. FENCES
   F. Bruen
3. I AM THE ENTERTAINER
   B. Joel
4. I CAN'T LOVE YOU ENOUGH
   B. Ellison
5. SEANCE
   R. Achilles

**SIDE TWO**

1. WATERMELON IS A KING'S DELIGHT
   R. Achilles
2. Y'ALL PUT YOUR SHOES ON
   B. Ellison
3. WORTH THE TIME
   R. Achilles
4. I NEVER MADE IT IN THE FIFTIES
   F. Bruen
5. SORRY, WE'RE CLOSED
   B. Ellison

"...If we could carve our work upon a stone,
And have it last throughout the ages,
Or enter words on eternal scrolls
With the sands of time upon the pages;
Still we'd dream of more to say
And think of different things to do
To share a moment as it happens,
We simply sing **OUR SONGS, FOR YOU...**"

*FAB COMPANY*

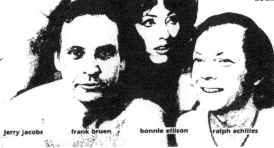

**jerry jacobs**    **frank bruen**    **bonnie ellison**    **ralph achilles**

## *We Live as We Can*

*© 1982 Bonnie Ellison / All Rights Reserved*

*Is there a reason for living?*
*Is there a goal to achieve?*
*A simple lesson of learning,*
*The love that we each need?*

*Is there a reason or purpose,*
*For creation of man?*
*We live, not as we wish to,*
*We live as we can.*
>*How can I tell you where I have been,*
>*Fighting a battle with fear?*
>*I believe there's a reason,*
>*For each of us here.*

>*I will sing a song of love,*
>*I'll sing my song for you.*
>*Each day is a new day.*
>*Make a new dream come true.*

*Is there a reason for dying?*
*Leaving the others behind?*
*I guess we'll just have to wait.*
*Our questions are answered by time.*

*I thought this happened to others.*
*"Why me?" I asked myself.*
*I don't need riches and fame,*
*Just give me my health...*

*Chorus*

*Is there a reason or purpose,*
*For creation of man?*
*We live not as we wish to,*
*We live as we can.*

*"We live not as we wish to, but as we can" quotation by Menander*

# VIII

## Eighth Month

## June

Time is a strange thing. It seems that we go through life always needing more of it, and never satisfied because of its limitations. It allows us to gain more knowledge and understanding with age and to recognize what we should have done at an earlier age. Like MS, time is also highly variable. It can last forever or, somehow, seem to pass us by.

Time for me was moving very slowly. I had lost control of half of my body. Physical impairment is frightening... mental impairment is worse. I had been through physical therapy in an effort to regain the use of my muscles and I had experienced mental confusion and depression which I was unable to cope with. The miraculous creation of my life had been altered and my living had temporarily been only existing.

Now, I look back and acknowledge the miraculous changes which have occurred, and I am thankful... to whom, I'm not sure. (But I never was very good at names...) I'm thankful to whomever or whatever was directing the course of my life. The intricate design of my life had been jarred out of place and I was left helpless. All of my human capabilities became meaningless. I felt as though I were a mere pawn whose direction was not my choice. My helplessness cannot be explained in words.

This personal frustration can best be explained with a line from a poem written by a friend of mine, Dr. David Luck: "If only I could speak out loud of what I feel within, I don't know how I'd tell you... where I have been."

Doctors can examine, diagnose, or identify a problem. They can prescribe drugs, which seem to help or reduce the pain or affect the mind, but there is so much more to be learned and they can only continue to try.

I experienced so much, while desiring so much more. I wanted an instant cure. My patience improved, but I still had a long way to go. At eight months, I could now walk normally, most of the time, and I had regained the full use of my right hand and arm. And now, I had proven to myself that I could even drive.

Eight months had passed since my attack, eight of the slowest months of my life. I had been through eight months, which seemed like eight years. I felt as though I'd had MS for most of my life, but now, at last, my old normality seemed within reach. Yet, so much had happened that it became difficult for me to remember my lifestyle before my attack.

My concern about my condition had seemed to erase most of my entertainment desires. My recuperating period had prevented me from seeing other entertainers perform. I really didn't want to see them. I was trying to accept the fact that I would never entertain again, and I didn't wish to rekindle any old desires. I felt as though I had admirably conquered my unrealistic dreams.

And yet, I couldn't help finding myself using my disease as an excuse. If only I had been given a chance to continue…

I found myself trying to hold back the tears after watching an exciting performance of an entertainer on television. And, finally, I found myself avoiding television entirely. I didn't need anything which prompted self pity.

But still, deep inside, I needed to be close to music, so I began devoting my time towards self education of the music industry and particularly, country music.

But there seemed to be a widespread misunderstanding common to my friends and relatives. It seemed that they expected me to relate all of the mysteries of life and the personal confrontations which I experienced through my songs. I had been where others had not. What did I see? Did I reach new meaningful conclusions in my life? Had I written any new songs?

## <u>Sorry, We're Closed</u>

*Sorry we're closed,*
*Said the sign on the door.*
*Only I could find a closed café,*
*Advertizin' open 24 hours a day.*

*Please come back again.*
*Sorry we're closed.*
*I'm tired and I'm hungry and I'm out of gas*
*And the station says sorry they're closed.*
> *If I ever get to Heaven,*
> *I don't expect to stay.*
> *There'll be a sign on the pearly gates*
> *Sayin' sorry, we're closed today*

*Sorry we're closed,*
*Everybody's gone home.*
*They may be sorry but it don't help me none,*
*Sorry never got nothin' done.*
> *If I ever get to Heaven,*
> *I don't expect to stay.*
> *There'll be a sign on the pearly gates*
> *Sayin' sorry, we're closed today.*

# IX

## Ninth Month

## July

I felt capable of writing "serious country". Maybe it's because I'm a Leo. I'm not saying that Leos are natural born country music writers, but they generally think they are capable of accomplishing all...

In this particular age, it is very important what astrological sign you are. The path of the principal planets, the moon, and the sun are represented by a band which is divided into twelve equal divisions or signs. Leo is the fifth sign of the zodiac.

Your sign is determined by your date of birth. Anyone who was born between July 23 and August 23 is a Leo. My Leo birthday is August 19.

Astrologers have supposedly identified particular characteristics which seem generally common to people who share the same sign. Leos are characterized as "born leaders, bold, energetic, weakness for flattery, ambitious and fickle", I'm not so sure about the "fickle" part, but the rest sounds pretty close to me.

It had been nine months since my MS attack. I had fully regained the use of my hand, my arm, and my leg, and I seemed to be mentally normal. I appeared normal physically. Mental adjustment was not as apparent.

I still had reminders of my hidden disease, though. I experienced intermittent problems: depression, lack of inspiration, right arm and shoulder aching, pressure on my temples, awareness of my heart beat, and some sleeplessness. Some nights, I seemed too hyper. I just couldn't seem to settle down. My right leg also occasionally felt tired and ached behind the knee.

My body seemed to experience a delayed reaction to what Dr. Ginsburg called my "overdoing it". Emotional upsets or such things as an overzealous hike would affect me the following week. I don't understand the relationship between physical activity and mental depression, but I did understand the fact that it occurred. The delayed effect of my activity made it extremely difficult for me to determine where the invisible line which distinguished "overdoing it" should be drawn. Trial and error seemed to be my only testing ground. It seemed strange to be testing my own body. How much could it endure? How much did it demand?

But time stands still for no one, depressed or elated, disabled or able… I had exercised both physically and mentally. I now knew more about the business of music than I ever did before and now I had an opportunity to listen to music more openly, determining popular commercialism.

I had even written some country material and had continued to play my guitar and sing. But my practice sessions were not always encouraging. I still enjoyed singing and I was thankful for regaining the ability and the physical movement to play the guitar again, but singing for my self enjoyment was totally different from performing for others. I had listened to me before…

I guess I missed the audience, the approval, the reassurance and the praise. Maybe that's why some people are entertainers. Maybe they need acknowledgement to justify the things which they desire. Maybe we all depend on acceptance by others to determine our way. So, I continued to practice.

I realized my own secret desires to perform, but I also recognized the nervousness inside of me which increased with the awareness of my heart pounding. As if that weren't enough, I had developed a new complex… I was afraid of people.

I, the Entertainer, was afraid of people! And I didn't even know why… I couldn't find any rational explanation for my fear. I could only attribute it to the mental changes and the helpless feelings which I seemed unable to control. So, I made a conscious effort to avoid people. This was something totally new. I couldn't believe it! I… the sarcastic, confident, outspoken female, the woman's libber… I was afraid of people…

But time seems to cure most ills, and time was good to me. I was eventually able to confront my fear more realistically and regained enough confidence to want to see other performers.

## The Night Belongs to the Entertainer

Walk along the street some night,
When its cold and dark,
When a cigarette flickers out
At the end of a spiraling arc.

That's the time to add up the day,
Think, and wonder, and there's nothing to say,
No-one to sing to, no-one to laugh,
The night belongs to the entertainer.

Hey entertainer, where are you going?
Hey entertainer, who's watching you now?
Not that sleepy old moon, way up in the sky,
Nobody's watching you now.

Hey entertainer, what are you doing?
Hey funny man, get rid of that frown
Her name is Bunny, pretty little Bunny.
Hey entertainer, let's blow this town.

City streets, rainy streets,
Beckoning to moonbeams.
Everyone's sleeping now,
Reckoning with new dreams.

Concert in Buffalo,
Club in Miami,
No use in hangin' 'round
For things that could never be.
City streets, rainy streets,
Beckoning to moonbeams.
The night belongs to the entertainer
So he can... dream his dreams.

Written in 1964 before the author started his life as an entertainer. It was prophetic.
Recoding history: Stylist Records, F.A.B. Company 1, 1970
From THE FUNNY ONE Ralph Achilles

# X

## Tenth Month

## August

Building confidence isn't easy. I needed all the help that I could get. Since it was summer, I decided that a nice, deep, dark tan couldn't hurt my ego. If I was going to make an effort to meet people, I at least wanted to appear healthy... even if I wasn't.

I had questioned Dr. Ginsburg about the effects of the sun on MS patients. I was told that patients seem to have more trouble during the summer months. They complain about the heat bothering them, making them tired and weak. People with MS seem to be affected by hot baths also. I had heard of patients becoming so weak that they were unable to get out of the tub.

Dr. Ginsburg asked me if I was a dedicated sun bather. I responded with the fact that I hadn't been before, but due to my inability to do much, plus my lack of energy, I felt that there was a good chance I might become one. This type of inactivity seemed as though it were designed for me. It took no effort and offered an opportunity to sleep and acquire a healthy looking bronze color change.

I've often wondered who originally decided that laying out in the sun in uncomfortable heat to end up with an uncomfortable sunburn, with the intention of slowly changing to a darker color rather than peeling, who decided that this darker color looked healthy or appealing? In an effort to be more appealing, most people end up just peeling!

Dr. Ginsburg suggested that I avoid the sun somewhat and not get burned. He actually wasn't that restrictive. He suggested that I begin my tanning by laying out about 10 or 15 minutes each day, to see how the sun affected me. He reminded me again that each MS person is different and that it had not been proven that the sun is harmful.

So it was again left up to me... All I knew was that 10 or 15 minutes a day in the sun for the rest of my life wouldn't produce a noticeable tanning effect on my body. I've always been envious of people whose skin turns a deep, dark brown from the sun. I can get tan, but I never achieve that dark, desirable, Coppertone color. So, 10 or 15 minutes a day to me meant virtually nothing.

But the fear of lying out in the sun and not being able to get back up did mean something, so I limited my first day of sunbathing to 15 minutes as directed. It seemed to have no effect... on either my tanning or my health. I felt fine but unfortunately, I didn't appear any tanner.

The next day, I tried 30 minutes. Again, I had the same results as the day before. The following day, I decided that I might as well do a little test run to determine how much my body could take.

I continued to increase my sunbathing time in an effort to appear healthy. After a period of time, I achieved my height of "brownness" with only minimal health effects, but there were some... My vision became very blurry after hours in the sun. I also experienced some tiredness and momentary visual blackouts when I'd get up too quickly.

But, people were telling me I looked great! My tan compensated for my minor sun problems. At least, I could still get up! The first few days, I would lie out for my limited time and then slowly try to move, expecting the sun to have paralyzing effects on me, but, if I could get up, I laid back down to get some more sun.

I was soaking up a little sunshine at Aunt Betty's condominium pool when I was surprised to see a familiar face, a fellow entertainer.

He was definitely wearing less than the last time I had seen him... but then again, so was I...

From our conversation, I learned that he lived in the same development and that he was now doing a single act, performing at a club nearby, called Brocks. He seemed very enthusiastic about working as a single, and soon was encouraging me to continue to entertain. He brought back a lot of old memories...

I tried to explain my mental fears, my nervousness, the difficulty I had in remembering the words to the songs, my lack of confidence as a single, but apparently, I wasn't very convincing. In a last effort to encourage my return to the stage, he offered me the use of his tape recording unit, for me to practice with until I regained my confidence. Not only did he offer the tape recorder, but he suggested that I use his microphone and his Ovation guitar which had an electrical input directly into the tape recorder.

Now, how could I pass this up! For each of my excuses, he offered a possible alternative. Why should he bother to encourage me? At least, why should he go out of his way, offering the use of his expensive equipment, trying to inspire me to continue to entertain?

I wasn't sure what he expected from me, but I accepted his offer... to borrow his equipment. My acceptance was rather indefinite as I thanked him, promising to go out to see him perform. I would have gone anyway. He didn't need to lure me with promises. Thank you Gary Morris.

I was interested in seeing Gary's show. Brocks offered him a small room with a comfortable, intimate atmosphere. He chose a very personal approach to his audience with the sincere honesty which typified his Texas upbringing.

I totally enjoyed his performance... his professionalism.

I was recognized in the audience. Gary introduced me over the microphone as Bonnie Lynne Ellison of the F.A.B. Company. The audience responded by applauding their support of our group. It felt great! It's always comforting to be accepted.

Then he asked if I would sing... I declined, but was thankful that he had offered.

After the show, several people stopped me to ask about the F.A.B. Company. I had secretly hoped that I wouldn't be recognized. I avoided any disease discussions and merely told them that Frank and Jerry were working in Kansas City and I was home, writing music. They must have accepted the fact that I had retired at the age of twenty-five or thought that I was hung up on writing at home.

Their next question was always the same. "Are you singing?" My answer was short, disguising the hurt: "No".

What was I doing? Nothing. But isn't that everyone's desire: to lay out in the sun all day and then be entertained at night? Who wants to work!

Somehow, it seems that everyone desires the unattainable, maybe everyone needs something to complain about. I had what ordinarily would be considered an ideal situation. I was happily married, I had lots of time, and I didn't need to work.

And yet, I had nothing to accomplish, nothing to achieve, nothing to replace my plans and dreams, which my health condition had interrupted. I know I could have found something but I wasn't interested in alternative courses in life. I needed time... more time to adjust to where I was, with what I had.

I didn't sleep well that night. The excitement of the club situation was destined to continue throughout the night for me. I couldn't turn the music off! For hours, I lay in bed, reliving Gary's show. I was envious of him; I wanted to sing. I wanted to, but I couldn't begin to face the real situation... the audience. I was frightened, too frightened to perform, but still desiring to relive the old memories, the emotional experiences.

I lay in bed, trying to convince myself of the ridiculousness of my new found fear. I had been on the stage since I was 12, in seventh grade, and performing professionally for the past five years! Now, I was afraid of people. The fact that I was unable to make myself face my fears was even more discouraging than any inability to perform.

But Gary's show had been inspiring. I promised myself that I would practice again, something which I had been neglecting. Maybe with time and practice, and more time, I would someday be able to perform again, to face an audience. At least the thought comforted my frustrations and allowed me to sleep... for that night...

# *Take Time*

*© 1973 Bonnie Lynne Ellison / All Rights Reserved*

*Take time to sit down and listen to me
I have something that I'd like to say.
'Though you may have heard it before,
I'd like to tell you in my own way.*

*I believe in people, do you?
I believe that the animals have souls too
I believe in warm nights and Creation in Spring.
I wonder if some believe in anything?*

*Do you think you believe in elves?
Do they play in the forest, in the leaves of the Fall?
Do you think you believe in yourself?
I wonder if some, ever think at all...
    (chorus)
I believe in Jesus, do you?
I believe in contentment, too.
I believe in Mother Earth, and the Heavens above.
I wonder if some still believe in love?*

*Take time to sit down and listen to me.
I have something that I'd like to say.
But nobody takes time to listen,
Everyone's busy today...*

I began practicing the next day. I made a list of the songs that I could perform and noted the key where I could best sing each of them. I even devised a practice show plan with the songs placed in a particular order for what I considered to be my best presentation. I envisioned trying to create a particular mood and then changing the pace with a subject or tempo variation. I changed the key for several songs, keys which had been chosen for the best trio voicing.

Looking over possible songs made me realize how limited my solo repertoire was. It was limited and old, but I do remember hearing, "There's no such thing as an old song... there's just old people." It generally contained songs which I had sung five years ago, before entering the F.A.B. Company.

I had to start somewhere! It was even enjoyable to go back to those old tunes and do a little reminiscing about my solo days before our group, but memories tend to exaggerate the good times and minimize the struggles, and there seems to be a great deal of distance between memories and reality. But, I practiced on! In a self-satisfying effort, I felt as though I was at least doing my best, beginning to confront my fears.

It had been about a week since I had seen Gary last, but he was back at the pool. He asked if I had been practicing. I told him that I had and expressed my enjoyment of his show. But, this time, he wouldn't let me change the subject away from practicing. This time, he was more demanding in offering his equipment. He gave me a specific time when I could pick it up, told me how long it would be available, and even offered to deliver it for me. That took care of any hesitancy on my part.

Arrangements were made. I now had Gary's sound system, his tape recorder, his microphone with stand, and his new electric Ovation guitar to use for three days and unlimited future availability.

The system was great! This was my first opportunity to even sing through a microphone since I'd had my MS attack. I was in Heaven! The system had a reverberation channel which sounded like an echo chamber. Now I could sit in the confinement of a small room and sing through the microphone, sounding like I was in Madison Square

Garden! I felt like I was home again… not Madison Square Garden, but behind a microphone. And I loved it!

There seems to be something very strange about entertainers. Something which may not be visibly detectable to others, drives you on and won't let go of you. That "something" had gotten me. The desire to entertain was inside of me. The need to entertain is habit-forming and I was definitely hooked. Withdrawal can be painful, regardless if it's a physical withdrawal or a mental one… a withdrawal from drugs or from a dream…

My excitement about singing was only dampened by my physical condition. My MS seemed to be catching up with me again. I received Gary's equipment on Monday. The previous weekend, I had felt so good that I had decided to take a hike while visiting our land, the 60 acres that Bob and I were buying. My little walk consisted of five hours of climbing either straight up a mountain or down a mountain and acted as another example of what Dr. Ginsburg meant by "overdoing it". I felt terrible for the next week. My right leg started things off by feeling tired again. Then it also decided to ache behind the knee.

The next day, my back became jealous of the competition, and it also decided to ache. This was accompanied by the return of the old pressure on the temples symptom. This continued throughout the week with additional tiredness, depression, lack of inspiration and energy. These MS side effects lasted until the following Tuesday when I began to feel more regular again.

So, my timing was very poor. I felt good, took my hike, and then felt bad during the time when I had Gary's equipment. I had trouble remembering the words to songs and it seemed that whenever I became nervous, I would blank out, totally forget the entire song, both the music and the words. I seemed to be doing fine as long as I was singing only for myself, but I became nervous even when one member of my family would listen. I was frustrated with myself and not feeling my best.

But the system did sound good. I pushed myself to practice.

August was here again; the only month when I age a whole year in a day.

I have a special day circled in my diary during this month; August 2. According to my notations on that day, I practiced my singing, my back had a tingling sensation, aching some, and I went to the library checking on books, which were available about MS.

I ended up not checking anything out, but going home to find that I had received a letter from an entertainment friend of mine, Anne Worcester. This letter was particularly meaningful to me. She asked if she could sing two of my songs in her shows.

I was excited... excited because someone liked my songs, and excited because she wanted to do them! This was my ultimate compliment; another professional singer offering to extend something which I had created.

Bob and I went out to dinner that night. I ran into Barb, a girl I had known in high school. (I couldn't remember her last name: 50% was great!) She asked me a question which is generally accepted as an old saying or greeting, "How's life treatin' you?" It definitely had more meaning now.

How's life treatin' me? Over twenty-five years had passed in my life, a quarter of a century, yet it seemed to me that I had experienced more than a lifetime. I could now stand up by myself. I could walk and talk. I could see and hear, feel and move. And, I could think again... and maybe, just maybe, I could write music, songs that others could relate to, or enjoy, or just share.

"Fine," I replied, smiling to myself. "Really fine..."

My circled day wasn't over yet. Bob and I had planned to meet Aunt Betty and her daughter and husband over at Brocks to listen to Gary sing that evening.

Following a few after dinner drinks, Bob and I were on our way. I was really "on my way". By now, I was feeling "really, really fine!" At least, I was all smiles. Alcohol has a tendency to make smiling easier.

We arrived at Brocks a little late, but a lot happier. Aunt Betty, cousin Sharon, and John were seated in front of the room full of people and had saved just enough room for Bob and I to join them. Gary was on the stage. I was just smiling…

Before Gary's break, he encouraged everyone to stay, promising the special appearance of a "real entertainer" during his next set. I anxiously wondered who was there and started looking around the room, to see whom I might recognize. When I couldn't find any local personalities, I thought that we might be in for a real treat. I assumed that our surprise entertainer was in the other room. I knew that it wasn't unusual for celebrities to be passing through town and agree to perform with the help of a little alcohol and coaxing. Whoever it was, I knew that I was glad to be there too.

Gary sang his closing song. You could hear a pin drop. The audience responded with strong applause as he left the stool where he'd been singing. He turned his microphone off, and walked directly over to the couch where I was sitting. Then he stopped, looked at me, and asked, "You will sing, won't you?"

# *I'm a Star*

*Your momma used to be in a band you know.*
*She was on the road, travellin' all around.*
*Then your daddy came along and touched my soul*
*And somethin' made me want to settle down.*

*I've never been to Nashville or to Hollywood.*
*I've never had a record playin' on the radio.*
*But I keep writin' songs for someone else to do.*
*They can go to Nashville, I'd rather be with you.*

*Me, I don't have to go far,*
*'Cause when I'm home with you,*
*I'm a Star. (repeat)*

*Momma's little baby's growin' up,*
*And I'm afraid that soon you'll be gone.*
*Why do the years keep getting' shorter?*
*It seems like the good times don't ever last long.*

*Me, I don't have to go far,*
*'Cause when I'm home with you,*
*I'm a star. (repeat)*

*Sometimes I get to thinkin' 'bout the band you know.*
*And the road starts lookin' awful good.*
*Then your daddy comes along and you smile at me,*
*And I'm content to be a star, in my neighborhood.*

*Me, I don't have to go far,*
*'Cause when I'm home with you, I'm a star.*
*Sophie, I don't have to go far*
*'Cause when I'm home with you, I'm a star.*

*I'm a well known, local celebrity singin' and a pickin' my guitar.*
*I don't need to go to Nashville or to Hollywood,*
*'Cause when I'm home with you, I'm a star.*
*When I'm home with you, I'm a star.*

# XI
## MS is...

I have Multiple Sclerosis (MS). I am 26 years old and share my incurable disease with "approximately 400,000 other people in the United States and 2.5 million people worldwide," according to the National Multiple Sclerosis Society. My initial attack came unexpectedly. No one expects a disease. One only learns to accept it . . .

Multiple Sclerosis is defined as a degenerative disease of the central nervous system. Degenerative means that there is a deterioration or a loss of function of the cells involved. It concentrates on the central nervous system, the brain and spinal cord, which is essential for directing nerve impulses throughout the body. MS often progressively gets worse with time. My disease may affect almost any part of the central nervous system, affecting almost any part of my body.

MS has been called "the enemy of young adults." Young people between the ages of 20 to 35 are prime victims of the disease. Although these are the years when initial symptoms generally appear, the disease can still occur in people anywhere from 18 to 40 years of age, and occasionally does, even before and after that time.

Young or old, MS is a proponent of equal rights and equal opportunity for all. Yet, there is a slight sexual discrimination with the disease, favoring women over men (2-3 to 1), and it does seem to have a preference for cold, damp climates. At least there are more patients in these areas. Moving to a warmer climate has not proven to be helpful. Unfortunately, Colorado has one of the highest MS diagnosis rates in the nation.

There doesn't seem to be an "average" type of MS case. Everyone is different . . . Variance within an individual and between patients often makes it difficult to even diagnose the disease to begin with. I was told not to compare myself to other patients, but it's only natural to be interested in other people who share the same disease. I found that patients vary from those who are completely paralyzed to others who are normal or near normal. Then, there are various degrees of severity in between. Naturally, it makes me wonder which type I may have, but progression of the disease cannot be predicted. Only time will give the answers.

I have lived with the awareness of my disease for only a short time, but it doesn't take very long to realize the constant changes which occur with MS. Reoccurring attacks known as exacerbations, or relapses, are interspersed with periods of partial or complete recovery known as remissions. It is therefore possible to be paralyzed during an exacerbation and then to regain normal use again during the remission phase of the disease. The improvement or recovery of a patient may be dependent on the degree of damage to a substance called myelin.

Nervous fibers or tracts in the brain and spinal cord are wrapped in myelin, a white fatty material or sheath which protects the fibers and helps conduct nervous impulses. When the myelin is damaged or destroyed, demyelination, nervous impulses are disrupted, interrupting messages from the brain. When only the myelin sheath is diseased, the nervous fiber may still be able to transmit some impulses, only with less strength.

There is no regeneration of myelin in the central nervous system. But patient recovery is recognized as inflammation is reduced in the area affecting the central nervous system. This improvement is called the remission period of the disease, but if the sheath is destroyed and the nervous tract is severely damaged or killed, nervous impulses cannot be carried, the nervous fibers cannot be restored, and permanent paralysis may result. Still, there is the possibility that if an area is not functioning, the body may bypass that area relying upon other nervous fibers for a relearning process.

Disability from the disease does not result from a problem in the muscle tissue, but from a faulty nerve pattern caused by demyelination. As the reoccurrence of exacerbations increases, the recovery from diseased areas becomes less complete.

When the myelin is broken down, scar tissue forms, leaving

patches of hardened tissue throughout the brain and spinal cord. The word "sclerosis" means hardening in Greek. Since the disease can affect more than one, or multiple parts of the central nervous system, and because it is also multiple exacerbations, it is called Multiple Sclerosis.

The exacerbations in MS are very unpredictable. Some people have been known to have only one attack while others may experience continuous problems. The number of exacerbations, the average length of each attack, and the amount of remission time between attacks is dependent on the individual patient.

There is not a specific test that always identifies Multiple Sclerosis. This explains the wide variation of patients who are diseased. Estimates have ranged from 250,000 to 500,000 MS patients in the U.S. alone. Other countries are not immune (approximately 2.5 million patients worldwide). Diagnosis is dependent on results of numerous tests - ruling out other possible problems - changes in the course of the disease, and a combination of individual symptoms which together may indicate Multiple Sclerosis. An MRI, magnetic resonance imaging, is ordered to view images of the brain and spinal cord, looking for lesions, or injuries, characteristic of MS. Having one or more of the symptoms does not indicate presence of the disease. Only a trained physician is capable of making a proper diagnosis.

The cause of Multiple Sclerosis is unknown. This leaves the field wide open for theorists. Everything from heredity, injury, virus, and allergy to vitamin deficiencies and psychological factors has been suggested, and these are only a few. It seems to me that for every theory I find, there's another theory with an opposing idea.

Since the cause is not known, treatment of the disease becomes more difficult. Advocates of theories tend to follow the treatment that is suggested depending on their choice of opinions.

Numerous drugs are also being used as treatments for Multiple Sclerosis in an effort to relieve the symptoms of the disease and to counteract its complications, but the erratic course of MS makes it difficult to determine the effectiveness of any particular treatment.

Some patients improve without any treatment. Others may benefit from treatment. No one is certain. Only statistical evidence of overall patients' improvement and the individual patient's response to a certain treatment can guide the physician's decision in prescribing medication.

Everything about Multiple Sclerosis is changeable! Therefore, it is not surprising to find varying degrees of severity in the disease. An acute type of MS may last only a few weeks or months, culminating in death, while other types may seem to disappear completely and may not significantly disable or shorten the patient's life.

Generally, the disease is characterized by a slow progressive downhill course leading to disability and ultimately death. Since all life must end in death, this course is not as shocking as it may first appear. It's the uncertainty of the disease which becomes frustrating. But even those without a disease are unable to predict the future.

A statistical average of the duration of the disease beginning from clinical onset of signs has been computed as 9 to 27 years, and yet this average figure tells very little because of the wide variation of the disease. There are MS cases that have been recorded which lasted from 40 to 60 years. So far, I have only been able to eliminate one type of MS for myself: I've lived longer than a few months since my diagnosis.

My disease was determined a year ago. I was told that most people with MS lead a near normal life. At that time, I wondered what "near normal" actually meant, but it didn't sound very drastic. And, since I hadn't even decided what a normal life was, I wasn't overly concerned about the change.

My life had been abnormal for years. I was a professional entertainer, so I felt like I had nothing to lose. I think that most entertainers are born only "near normal" to begin with…

Since my initial exacerbation, I have now recovered back to my "near normal" condition. Presently, I am in a remission stage. Outwardly I appear very normal. My disease is undetectable. Only I am aware of the symptoms which persist, the varying tiredness, lack of inspiration and energy, physical aches, visual problems, and equilibrium difficulties.

My life has changed during the past year. I have experienced both paralysis and recovery, and the questions, fears, and frustrations of a disease which I had never heard of before.

But I found that my ignorance was not uncommon. Neither my

family nor my friends were very knowledgeable about Multiple Sclerosis. It seemed to me that everyone knew someone who had MS, but no one was certain what the disease was or how it actually affected the patient.

As time continued I discovered that my personal experiences were not as unique as I had originally expected. I wasn't alone... Many others shared my same concerns and misunderstandings. I cannot offer answers. I can only share my own personal experiences and impressions. Something may sound familiar. But then again, especially with MS, everyone is different.

# Life Is Just a Puff of Dreams

*(spoken)*
*"The night that the old man died,*
*All the rivers whispered.*
*It seemed as though the world stood still,*
*As he struggled to be heard.*

*And I was such a little boy*
*And he so very old.*
*I'll always feel an inner pride,*
*It was me the old man told."*

*(song)*
    *Life is just a puff of dreams,*
    *That winks and fades away.*
    *Before you taste a buttercup,*
    *The petals all turn to clay.*

    *Listen to the carousel,*
    *That calls you to the fair.*
    *Search not for the pot of gold*
    *But the rainbow shining there.*

    *Only when you turn around,*
    *You truly understand.*
    *For the sparkle of an instant,*
    *You held a snowflake in your hand.*

*And though we have to fight,*
*To make a newer dawn,*
*It's the love within the moment,*
*That makes the truth live on.*

    *Repeat (song)*

# XII

## Twelfth Month

## October

Multiple Sclerosis taught me lessons of life. Dreams and memories come and go unexpectedly. My dreams had faded away and my memories were lost. I learned how helpless I was. I was not in control. I learned to "wait". I learned about acceptance and about patience, how to cope and hope.

As I battled the extremes of my disease, the highs and lows, mental confusion and physical weakness, I learned that I couldn't rely on my body, or my mind, to stay the same. Everything changed constantly. I didn't know what to expect next. I couldn't plan an hour, a day, or a dream. I couldn't plan my future under such volatile conditions. I learned to be afraid of the future, to fear change. I later realized that, without change, there is no progress.

When I was fortunate enough to regain the use of parts of my body and my mind, I learned to be grateful. I simply learned that "When you've got your health, you've got it all!"

I felt weak, angry, and afraid. I had no answers, and couldn't even remember my questions. No one could depend on me, and I couldn't even depend on myself. I was shaken. I had no base. From that, I learned about depression, low self-esteem, and paranoia. I also learned acceptance of others, to reject self-pity, and to have a little faith.

I was thankful for my recovery, but nothing was assured. I learned to be thankful. I learned about gratitude. Like the song said, I was "walking on broken glass." My life had been shattered.

Now, I understand Achilles' song, "Life is Just a Puff of Dreams." There are no assurances in life. You can lose everything in a few seconds. We need to live, enjoying each day, living now, not always projecting our happiness into the future. We need to love each moment of truth.

As Achilles said, "for a sparkle of an instant, you hold a snowflake in your hand." We each touch miracles.

## <u>*Good Lovin' Man*</u>

### ©*2001 Bonnie Lynne Ellison / All Rights Reserved*

*I always wanted a cowboy . . .*
*A savior, on a white horse.*
*Someone to trust and believe in,*
*I'd surrender my love, of course.*

*I always wanted a cowboy . . .*
*Tight jeans, boots, and a hat,*
*Ridin' a horse, out on the range,*
*Livin' and lovin', wherever he's at.*

> *I always wanted a cowboy,*
> *Lean muscled, and ruggedly tan.*
> *I am sure, I got more,*
> *I got a good, lovin' man.*

> *Doo doo dooby doo dooby, doo doo dooby doo doo . . . .*

*He wanted to be, a cowboy.*
*A man, silent and strong.*
*Secure in his word, with a handshake,*
*Knowin' the difference, between right and wrong.*

*He wanted to be a cowboy,*
*He wanted to play a guitar.*
*Sing about cowpokes and gamblin',*
*Smokin', and drinkin', in a bar.*

> *Chorus*

*I always wanted a cowboy,*
*Someone to take care of me,*
*Satisfy my womanly needs,*
*Treat me like a lady . . . .*

*I always wanted a cowboy . . .*
*Dreamin' 'bout acres to roam,*
*He has a job, a truck, and a dog,*
*And we just can't stop, smilin' at home.*

> *Chorus*

148

40 years later...

# Reflections
**The National Little Britches Rodeo Association**
**August, 2010**

"I love the rodeo"... It will always be a part of me.

I remember carrying the American flag in the Grand Entry Parade. I remember the sound of my horse's hoofs pounding, mixed with speed, danger, and excitement, with the symbolic cloth flapping in the wind.

I remember the cowboy rodeo prayer, humbly asking for protection.

I remember the carnival, and the "carnies," with their sun parched skin and tattooed arms. The carnival smelled like cotton candy and had the romance of youth, the smell of perfume and cologne. I remember the brilliant, multicolored lights and colors, the sound of music and the sound of the carnival games, the rifles popping, the balloons bursting, the basketballs hitting the rims, and the "prizes," love offerings of huge, overstuffed bears.

I remember the sun, the incessant heat, and the dirt, the jeans and the boots, the chaps, and the jingling of spurs, the horse dander, the smell of hay, alfalfa, and Omolene... I remember the smell and the sound of the livestock, the cows bellowing, their bells ringing, and the smell of their natural fertilizer.

I remember the excitement of getting up at dawn "to feed," practicing events for hours, currying animals, carrying water pails, cleaning stalls with my pitchfork, sitting on fences, the thrill of winning, and the depression of a loss.

I remember the fear in the pit of my stomach, as I summoned up enough courage to compete in the life threatening events. The rodeo was my first recognition of danger.

I remember watching Cody, invincible at eight years old, when the enormous, big horned bull stepped on his face, after ejecting him. I remember the blood, the broken bones, the permanent scars, the paralysis, and near death challenges which resulted from the competition. Great confidence was gained by those young athletes who apparently wanted to win a saddle as much as I did.

The National Little Britches Rodeo Association is alive and well! The "rodeo for kids' started in 1952, and was held annually until 1961, when a national youth rodeo association was established. Today, the World Championship Finals for the junior rodeo are held in Pueblo, Colorado, at the Colorado State Fairgrounds. www.nlbra.com

"The Rodeo contestants have three age divisions, the Little Wranglers, the Junior Division, and the Senior Divisions.

The Little Wranglers are boys and girls, aged 5-7, who compete together in Flag Racing, Pole Bending, Barrel Racing, and Goat Tail Untying.

Contestants who are 8-13 years of age compete in the Junior Division. The Junior and Senior Divisions are divided into separate Girls and Boys categories. The Junior Girls compete in Trail Course, Barrel Racing, Pole Bending, Goat Tying, and Breakaway Roping. Junior Boys compete in Steer/Bull Riding, Bareback Riding, Flag Racing, Goat Tying, and Breakaway Roping. Girls and Boys compete together in the Junior Team Roping and the Daily Ribbon Roping.

The Senior Division is for contestants aged 14-18. The Senior Girls compete in Barrel Racing, Pole Bending, Trail Course, Goat Tying, and Breakaway Roping. Senior Boys compete in Bull Riding, Bareback Riding, Saddle Bronc Riding, Steer Wrestling, and Tie-Down Roping. In Team Roping, Senior Girls and Boys compete together.

I did it all! In the early years, in the 60's, the Senior Girls could compete in Bareback Bronc Riding. I was a Senior Girl, so I did it!

I remember the RCA cowboy who "set me down" on the horse, the "roslin' glove" to glue my hand onto the handle of the "riggin'" which was tied around the horse. We drew numbers for our buckin' horse. I was supposed to come out of the chute second. My horse was a full grown yearling who, at the time, was panicking... The horse kept rearing up and falling down in the chute. I straddled the horse with my feet on the gate and the fence, my heart pounding, both excited and scared to death…

There were only five young cowgirls in my event. Less competition! But my horse wouldn't settle down, so I was passed up from second to last. Right before me, the girl's horse ran straight across the arena and directly into the fence. She broke her leg, the contestant. The ambulance pulled up in the dirt, she was loaded up, they drove off, and then, it was my turn.

I sat down on the horse, laid back on his rear end as instructed, and then spurred the horse out of the chute, "marked" him on his first jump. After that, everything was in slow motion, like a movie. I laid back as far as I could, holding on to the riggin' with my right hand, the other hand held high in the air, but I was frightened when I couldn't see my horse's head. (Guess it must have been between his front legs.)

My horse ran to the center of the arena, and came to an abrupt stop as he planted both of his front feet into the dirt. Then he began bucking. I slowly felt like I was slipping down to the left side, still in slow motion. Each jolt was extreme when the horse came down on his front legs. I knew I was falling. Then my slow motion was jolted back to reality when my head hit the ground and I couldn't breath. I remember the horse's feet going over my head, so close.

I prayed that he'd miss me. The pick up men, picked me up, and finally I was able to breathe again. I was so thankful… I survived! Then, over the loud speaker, the announcer said that I was awarded a re-ride! Apparently I could hold on as well as anyone. I had pulled the riggin'over my horse's head. As far as a re-ride, I passed… This event was later eliminated in the rodeo, due to multiple injuries.

Little Britches is a lot safer now. Helmets, mouth guards, and protective vests are now used, but we must remember that "we're not in charge," especially when we're dealing with a dangerous sport, with wild animals that weigh 2,000 pounds.

Contestants have died. These terrible tragedies are rare and uncommon. Animals will do everything to avoid stepping on anything they perceive as not stable or unsafe. I guess "they're not in charge" either…

"I love the rodeo"... There is always music... and a big country dance. From Little Britches to the Greeley Stampede, to the National Western Stock Show, loud speakers, drums, guitars, bass, fiddles, and steel guitars fill the air.

I love the night-lights full of anticipation, the rides, the hot dogs, popcorn, balloons, feathers, caramel apples, the ferris-wheel, and the merry-go-round. I love the excitement of the personal competition, both in and out of the arena. I love the hats and the sweatin', the buckles, and the belts.

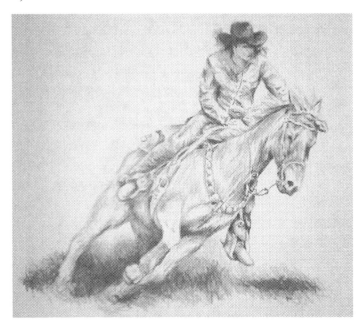

Achilles and Frank, and Jerry didn't rodeo, but they did have multiple talents.

Frank Bruen founded and operated Bruen Productions International, Inc. for radio and TV production. Today, he is an audio-video, WEBmercial producer: http://www.bruendirect.com

Ralph Achilles is a successful comedian, musician and singer performing on the Royal Caribbean and Celebrity Cruise Lines: http://www.ralphachilles.net. He is THE FUNNY ONE!

Jerry Jacobs, after 30 years, continues to be a successful Realtor with RE/MAX Southeast, Inc. www.jacobsteam.net. Jerry, a Lifetime Achievement Award recipient, established The Jacobs Team along with his son and daughter.

Gary Morris is an "International Award winning vocalist and actor, best known for his original recording of "The Wind Beneath My Wings" www.garymorris.com

They are truly the "Real Entertainers!"

I think that I've experienced every problem that you can with MS. Migraine headaches have been debilitating. But I've been fortunate. After several years, my disease was termed "stabilized," and I was able to regain my "near normality." I performed for Gary Morris, and continued to entertain with the F.A.B. Company, on a limited basis. I have been offered performance contracts in Las Vegas, and entertainment contracts with the William Morris Talent Agency. I've written, recorded, and heard my songs, on the radio at home and in my car. After TV appearances, radio interviews, indoor and outdoor concerts, standing ovations, and signing autographs, I went back to school. I got a degree in Elementary Education, got a Professional Teacher License, taught school, updated my Real Estate License to a Brokers License, and sold new homes.

Originally, I was told that I would never walk normally again, but I might regain the use of my right arm and hand. My philosophy is: Ignore negative information and never give up. I attribute my recovery to "early diagnosis", my doctors, the support of my family and friends, my competitive nature, my spiritual growth, and my daughter. I also believe in Sunlight for vitamin D, Oxygen for B12, Exercise for feeling good, Meditation for stress, and Caffeine for fatigue.

Now, I've taught school for over 20 years, I show new homes, and I write songs. I even joined NSAI (Nashville Songwriters Association International) and took my songs to Nashville. I'm still waiting...

I have lived with Multiple Sclerosis for almost 50 years. I always wanted to be a singer... my dream came true. Now I am closer to my God who guides me, comforts me, and takes care of me. He gives me words to say, songs to sing, and music to play.


Dad was right.

"When problems start showin', hitch up your buckle, and keep on goin'."

His problems started showin', at eighty-five, when he slipped and broke his leg, while exercising one of his horses. His "end of the trail" followed a downward progression of health problems and hospitals. After a year of struggling... his machines were turned off.

My dad, the man who was the strength of my life... the smartest... the funniest... the fastest runner... the best bowler... the best swimmer... the best golfer... the best dancer... the best horseman... my champion and my hero... raised both of his hands upward to the hospital ceiling, and unwillingly gave his final order, "Go ahead and take me... " Then, he quietly hitched up his buckle, and kept on goin'... forever.


I waited four years and then a miracle happened.

My baby had a baby, on my birthday. . . .
   Baby Savannah Vivian was born on August 19th.
      Now, Sophie is a mother, and Shane is a father. . . .

I'm a "Grandmother" and my mother is a "Great- Grandmother!"
   "The circle of life continues... "
      "We are truly miracles ... surrounded by miracles."

                  "Really, ... how can you not sing?"

# The Colorado Sky

Get under the covers, close your eyes,
Promise not to cry,
And your daddy will tell you the story
Of the Colorado sky.

Now, my son, the story starts
A whole universe away,
In a place where everybody laughs,
Just like we did today.

And oh Tony, the people there,
They'd never make you cry,
There's not a one that's mean, or cross,
And they never, never, lie.

For all these people live with God,
Like other people do,
And God loves all his children
As Mother and I love you.

Yes, some day, I'm sure you can
Go and live with Him.
For everyone who learns to love,
Gets to walk with him.

And while we wait to join him
He gives us golden land
And after we have planted it, he offers us his hand.

And all that ripened fruit
That we planted in the Fall,
Is left for those who follow us,
And wait to hear His call.

And just to make us feel
That He is always near,
He took some parts of heaven
And gave them to us here.

*He planted mighty Redwood trees*
*All along the sea*
*And orchards, deep with flowers,*
*As far as you can see.*

*But here, in Colorado,*
*Where His mountains stand so high,*
*He placed the perfect gift of all,*
*A piece of heaven's sky!*

*And oh Tony, its grand to see,*
*Its colors change all day,*
*It goes from red, to orange, to blue,*
*And never fades away.*

*Now get under the covers, close your eyes,*
*You'll see it, if you try,*
*God's gracious gift to us, my son,*
*The Colorado sky.*

*Recording History: Norman Records, Achilles and Frank, 1967, Pax Records,*
*Take Time, F.A.B. Company, 1971, Fall River Records, Achilles Solo Album,*
*1975. Iliad Publishing Co.*

"I have been from here to there, and back again.
Made decisions, erased by time.
But who am I to decide the Reason?
The answers that I find are only mine."


➢ *Bonnie Lynne Ellison*

# Glossary

**ACTH- (a)dreno (c)ortico (t)ropic (h)ormone** - Signals the body to produce more naturally to cope with stress.

**Auto immune disease** - The body attacks its own tissue.

**Caffeine** – a stimulant and diuretic.

**Central nervous system (CNS)**- The central nervous system is the brain and the spinal cord.

**Diets**- A person's regular food and drink. The National MS Society does not recommend any special diets for MS patients.

**Exacerbations**- Reoccurring attacks known as exacerbations, or relapses, are interspersed with periods of partial or complete recovery known as remissions, a worsening of symptoms.

**Exercises** – Physical or mental exertion to maintain fitness.

**Faith** – Religious beliefs.

**Fatigue** – Tiring or weakness.

**Friends** – People who one likes.

**Migraines** – Severe headache usually only on one side of the head with nausea.

**MRI (Magnetic Resonance Imaging)**- A test which can show plaques, scarring, and lesions caused by MS in the spinal cord.

**Multiple Sclerosis**- A degenerative disease of the central nervous system. Degenerative means that there is a deterioration or a loss of function of the cells involved. It concentrates on the central nervous system, the brain and spinal cord, which is essential for directing nerve impulses throughout the body. MS often progressively gets worse with time. MS disease may affect almost any part of the central nervous system, affecting almost any part of the body.

**Myelin-** A white, fatty substance surrounding nerve fibers.

**NDE (Near Death Experience)** – Same or similar experiences reported in near death instances.

**NLBRA (National Little Britches Rodeo Association)** - "The National Little Britches Rodeo Association is a youth rodeo for kids aged from 5-18.

**Optic Neuritis** – Inflammation of the optic nerve which connects to the eye, which connects to the brain.

**Pregnancy** – The time when women are carrying a developing fetus in their uterus.

**Prednisone** – Corticosteroid which is an anti-inflammatory homornal preparation.

**Remission** – Partial or complete recovery.

**Relapses-** Exacerbations or attacks.

**Societies** – Organizations of people interested in MS.

**Sun** – A star in our solar system which is the source of heat and light, the center of our planetary system.

**Tests** – A trial or proof.

**Vitamins-** Complex, organic substance essential for maintaining life.

# About the Author

Bonnie Lynne Ellison is an award-winning musician, vocalist, songwriter and teacher who has appeared on television and radio, in movies, and on the stage. She is a published writer, poet, entertainer, and Multiple Sclerosis patient.

She is the author of the MS series, 'MS Entertainer', published in the National Multiple Sclerosis Society's Northern Chapter in Fort Collins, Colorado. This is a patient's perspective of the disease, an excerpt from her book.

Bonnie and her entertainment group, the F.A.B. Company, held the first MS Radio-thon on KHOW to raise money for Colorado MS patient services.

Her first song, "I'm Young and Free," was published in the Young Women's Christian Association (YWCA) National Songbook when she was a Senior in high school.

Bonnie grew up in Littleton, Colorado. She played the drums at North Elementary School, electric guitar in the Jazz Band at Grant Junior High School, and won the Kiwanis Club Stars of Tomorrow Talent Show at Littleton High School. She "brought the house down" at Grant Junior High School's talent shows and at Colorado State University's Green and Gold Review during C.S.U's infamous College Days. She won Vocalist of the Year at Grant and continued to compete in talent shows at Littleton High School.

Bonnie performed at college in Ft. Collins as a soloist, playing her guitar, until she sang with Frank Bruen as "Frank and Bonnie". She later joined Achilles and Frank, the Internationally acclaimed entertainment duo, to form the F.A.B. Company, Frank, Achilles and Bonnie, which recorded and toured Nationally. Jerry Jacobs later joined the group as a musician and vocalist.

In 1973, Bonnie was diagnosed with Multiple Sclerosis, while performing in Olympia, Washington.

Her mission is to inspire hope for millions who are facing this unpredictable disease.

When she isn't writing, she teaches school. She resides in Littleton, Colorado, close to the mountains and her family.

Order Form

To order additional copies of **MS ENTERTAINER** books, go to Google. com and enter **MS ENTERTAINER**.

To order **F.A.B. Company** songs on CD and MP3 downloads, go to Amazon.com and search for **MS ENTERTAINER**.

**Thank you,**
**"The Tonight Show Starring**
**Jimmy Fallon."** ☺

A lot has changed since I was diagnosed with MS. Successful treatments, achievements, advancements, and new technology improve people's lives.

**The National Multiple Sclerosis Society** continues ongoing research to end this global disease.

"Nearly 1 million people (913,925)" are living with MS in the US in 2019.

Printed in the United States
By Bookmasters